Juicer Recipes

A Complete Juicing Guide on Juicing and the Juicing Diet

Helen Rauscher and Trena Tufts

Table of Contents

CHAPTER 5: YOUR 7 DAY JUICING DIET MEAL PLAN.88

SECTION 2: JUICING DIET 92

CHOOSING A JUICER 99

TRAVELING WITH JUICE 102

FRUIT-ONLY JUICES 103

Introduction

Why Go On A Juicing Diet?

One of the biggest benefits to the juicing diet is weight loss. Weight gain and excessive weight and fat account for many bad health issues. Juicing adds more benefits that just weight loss. You could look at weight loss as a side benefit to the other reasons for juicing. One of the best reasons to juice is to help cleanse the body of impurities. Some refer to this as a type of detox diet plan. While there are many diets that help with weight loss, many cannot claim the added benefit of detox. A juicing diet plan means that the recipes within this book can replace your needed daily water intake because juice contains plenty of water along with other healthy antioxidants and even fiber. While juicing diet alone can help to shed the weight and unwanted fat, it is not a super-fast process (no diet is). In order to make juicing successful you should couple it with a good exercise program. Exercising the body is very healthy and beneficial to the body.

Juicing is beneficial for your health with weight loss as a side benefit if you consider the other benefits. To use juicing for health reasons, weight loss included, you need to make a commitment to bring juicing into your lifestyle as well as diet plans. Incorporating juicing in the diet is like any other habit you form, it takes time to see results. Just like eating right all the time should be a lifestyle choice, juicing can be a lifestyle choice too.

Add Juicing To Your Dieting Lifestyle

While it may be fine to go on a strict juicing diet, it helps to incorporate it into your dieting lifestyle, because at some point you will want to eat solid foods. The fact that juicing provides a wonderful amount of nutrients should be enough reason to continue to juice in some ways on a daily basis.

If you are wishing to lose weight, then juicing is a great way to do so. Many different diets and even diet pills out there promise to help shed the unwanted fat. Most diet pills are just appetite suppressants. Instead of popping pills that may have bad side effects, you can try drinking juice, heavy with vegetables. Fresh vegetable juice is a natural appetite suppressant and so much healthier. It will help to give the stomach a full feeling, which helps you not to grab for more food. An effective way to use vegetable juice as an appetite suppressant is to drink a glass of vegetable juice a few minutes before a meal. You will not eat as much.

Fresh vegetable juice is also good for people with blood sugar issues as it helps to stabilize and normalize the blood sugar levels. Vegetable juice is naturally low in sugar. Vegetables are plenty sweet though in flavor which helps to satisfy a sweet tooth. If you get a craving for sweets try drinking a cup of vegetable juice and see if it does not satisfy the urge. The key to success in controlling blood sugars are to go lightly on the fruit juices and focus more on vegetables.

Weighing the Cost of a Juicing Diet

The first thing you will want to do when you decide to go on the juicing diet is to purchase a good juicer. You may find these to be pricey, but if you consider it an investment to your health, you will realize it is a good investment. Compare the cost of a juicer to the cost of specialty foods offered on certain diet plans. You will no doubt be saving money after that first initial purchase. The only thing you will have to purchase afterward will be the actual fruit and vegetables.

Using juicers are easy if you have a good brand. You will want your juicer to sit on your countertop because you will be using it daily. Buy a brand that is reputable and highly recommended.

Juicing Fasts and Just Juicing

If you are going to juice because you are overweight, you may want to consider doing a "juicing fast" where you fast from all solid foods and drink nothing but fresh fruit and vegetable juice. This gives you a twofold benefit, because in addition to helping lose unwanted weight and fat you are also doing a body cleanse. You are giving your body a break from all the additives in foods and allowing the natural nutrients found in fruit and vegetables to help clean out the inside of your body. It is beneficial for the liver, kidneys, blood, and the digestive system. Once you have jumpstarted the weight loss you can work juicing in with a healthy nutritious diet.

If pure vegetable juice is still not palatable to you try adding a fruit or two in the mix. You will be surprised at how the fruit will overpower the vegetables in flavor. On the other hand, try adding spices to your vegetable juice. Even a dash of salt and pepper will make all the difference. Even if you just drink one glass of vegetable juice a day with your healthy diet, you will see a noticeable difference in your general well-being. A glass of juice a day will help to strengthen the immune system, will aid with proper digestion, will get rid of water retention, and give you energy.

Exercising and Juicing

If you want to turbo charge your dieting you should add a good exercise routine with it. The fact is that the body needs exercise in order to be healthy. Even a juicing diet will go better if you are working out regularly. Just do simple half hour easy exercises every other day for the best results. Even walking will help. The point is to get the body to moving more. You will find the weight will fall off faster and you will have more energy. Always seek the advice of your physician first.

Section 1: Juicing Guide

More than likely, you have heard all about juicing and juicing diets. However, you may not be familiar with the truth about juicing, especially when it comes to juicing and weight loss. Many people try to start a juicing diet without actually learning what juicing is all about, how long they should being on a juice-only diet and the benefits that juicing has to offer.

If you have considered juicing for weight loss, this guide is for you. This juicing guide offers helpful information on juice, the benefits of juicing and so much more. You will even find some great tips that will make your juice diet even more successful. The best part about this juicing guide is that it is packed with the tastiest, healthiest juicing recipes out there. Whether you enjoy vegetable flavored juices or you like the sweeter juices, you are sure to find great recipes that will fit with your tastes and your lifestyle. Many of the recipes included are very easy to make, especially with the help of a quality juicer.

Do not start your juicing diet until you read this guide. With this guide by your side, you can begin juicing for weight loss, armed with important information and great recipes. Even when you stop juicing for every meal, you can go back to this guide for great juicing recipes that can be used anytime for a great dose of vitamins and minerals.

Chapter 1: What is Juicing?

Before you begin juicing for weight loss, it is important to know more about juicing and how it works. What is juicing? Juicing is simply defined as the process of extracting juices from vegetable of fruit plant tissues. Juicing can be done in several different ways. Some fruits can be juiced by hand, but to get the most juice from most fruits and vegetables, a good juicer is needed.

Many people choose to juice fruits and vegetables because it offers the body many important nutrients in a way that can easily be assimilated by the body. When juicing fruits and veggies at home with a domestic juicer, the produce is prepared and then pushed through the feeding chamber of the juicer. Then the machine uses either a separation or pureeing process to juice the produce.

In most cases, you do not need to peel produce before putting it through the juicer. However, some fruits and vegetables may be exceptions. For example, oranges and other citrus fruits happen to have bitter oils in their peels, which is why it is best to peel them before they are juiced. Fruits and vegetables with a very hard rind, such as squash, pumpkins, watermelon and other similar items of produce will need to have the peel or rind removed to avoid damaging the juicer.

One of the main reasons that juicing has become so popular is because taking in fresh, raw produce is actually much better than taking in vegetables that have been cooked. The juices help to remove toxins and waste from the body, also working to regenerate and repair body tissues. Fresh juices also provide plenty of important enzymes and antioxidants to the body, which can help to improve metabolism, help along metabolic processes and eliminate free radicals within the body.

Juicing not only helps to preserve the important nutrients found in veggies and fruits, but it also allows individuals to take in more produce at one time than they could if they were eating it. A large glass of fruit or vegetable juice includes the juice of more fruits and veggies than you could ever eat at one time.

Of course, while many people can definitely benefit from a juicing diet, it is always a good idea to talk to your doctor before starting any new diet. People who may be taking prescription medications or dealing with an illness need to talk to their doctor before drinking a large quantity of juice, since juices may change the way their body metabolizes the medications they are taking.

For most healthy individuals, juicing provides a healthy, safe way to begin increasing the intake of important nutrients. Even juicing for one meal a day can provide great results.

While some people choose to only juice for one meal each day, others decide to go on a juice diet for a few days where they only take in juices. This may be okay for a few days, but a diet of only juices is usually not a good idea for more than a few days at a time. For the best results, you can drink only juices for a few days and then you can go back to eating a regular healthy diet while drinking a glass of juice for one of your meals each day.

Chapter 2: Benefits of Juicing

Before you decide to start juicing for weight loss, you may want to take a closer look at the benefits juicing can offer you. Juicing has become quite popular because of the many benefits to it. Maybe you have heard other people talk about how great juicing is but wondered if it really can help you. Here is a look at some of the top benefits you can enjoy when you try the juicing diet yourself.

Benefit #1 – Efficiently Consume Large Amounts of Fruits and Veggies

One of the main benefits of juicing is that it allows you to efficiently consume large amounts of fruits and veggies. You should be getting more than five servings of fruits and vegetables each day. The problem is that most people never get that many servings of fruits and veggies. It can be difficult to fit all those fruits and veggies into your meals each day. However, juicing makes it a lot easier for you to get all the fruits and vegetables that your body really needs. In fact, you could actually get all the recommended servings of fruits and veggies in a single glass of juice. This makes it fast and convenient to begin adding more healthy produce to your life on a regular basis.

Benefit #2 – Include a Wide Variety of Fruits and Veggies in Your Diet

Another great benefit of juicing for weight loss is the ability to include a wide variety of fruits and veggies in your diet. If you are eating vegetables and fruits regularly, it is easy to get into a rut. Soon you may find that you are eating the same fruits and veggies on a regular basis. This means that you may not be getting the wide variety of vitamins and minerals that are needed by your body. When you begin juicing, you can include a wider variety of great fruits and veggies in your juices, making sure that you get a wide variety of different nutrients that your body needs.

Some people find that they do not particularly like the flavor of certain fruits and vegetables. When you begin juicing, you can enjoy the benefits of fruits or veggies you do not like as much without having to taste them. Many times you can add certain veggies or fruits to a juice with another fruit or vegetable that has a predominant flavor, overpowering the flavor of the item you do not like. You do not have to avoid certain veggies and fruits just because you do not like their flavor. You can easily add them to juices and get all their benefits without tasting them specifically.

Benefit #3 – Enjoy More Energy

One of the greatest benefits that people often notice after they begin juicing is that they enjoy more energy. One reason that you may experience more energy when juicing is because your body does not have to use very much energy to digest the veggie and fruit juices. The juicers are almost totally digested. You simply drink the juice and your body will not need to use much energy on digestion. Since you are saving all that energy, you will probably notice that your energy levels begin to increase.

Many people that do not get enough fruits and vegetables notice that they feel fatigued on a regular basis. If you are dealing with fatigue and the need to sleep more than usual, juicing may be able to help. After you begin juicing for a few days, you will quickly find that your energy levels begin to skyrocket, which can help improve your life in many different ways.

Benefit #4 – Get Plenty of Chlorophyll From Green Juices

Many of the juicing recipes that you will find in this juicing guide and in other places include produce that contains a lot of chlorophyll. You will especially find a large amount of chlorophyll in the greener juices that include a large amount of greens, such as spinach.

Chlorophyll is a great detoxifier and is found naturally in plants. When you begin getting more chlorophyll in your diet, you will find that it helps to eliminate parasites from the body. It also strengthens your body, helps to rebuild your blood cells and helps purify and detoxify your body as well.

Benefit #5 – Detoxify Your Liver for Better Health

You will also find that juicing for weight loss can offer the benefit of detoxifying your liver for better health. Your liver has so many functions that it has to undertake on a regular basis and these functions are very important to the way your body works. One of the most important functions of your liver is to clean out the blood, removing metabolic waste and toxins from the blood. Since most people end up being exposed to many toxins on a regular basis, the liver needs to be in great shape so it can keep your blood as clean as possible.

Some of the best antioxidants that help to cleanse out your liver include vitamin C, beta carotene and vitamin E. Niacin and various B vitamins also help to cleanse the liver as well. Some great veggies that are known to be good for detoxifying the liver include cauliflower, Brussels sprouts and cabbage. Adding some of these veggies to your juices from time to time can help ensure you enjoy this benefit from your juicing.

Benefit #7 – Enjoy Healthier, More Beautiful Skin and Hair

When you begin juicing on a regular basis, you can also enjoy healthier, more beautiful skin and hair. For many people, this benefit is unexpected. When you begin juicing, you will be able to increase your intake of veggies and fruits that contain vitamin E and vitamin C. Both of these vitamins work to help protect your skin from damage when it is exposed to the sun. Some of the best fruits to use to get these vitamins include blueberries and blackberries. In fact, you'll find some recipes in this juicing guide that combine blueberries and blackberries, which can help you get the vitamins you need for healthier skin.

If you are not getting enough riboflavin in your diet, you can experience hair loss, cracked lips and a variety of different skin problems. Some of the veggies that have a lot of riboflavin in them include spinach and kale, which are found in many of the juicing recipes included. As you begin getting more of this important vitamin, you will notice that your skin begins to get healthier and the hair loss problem may begin to abate as well. Many other vitamins and minerals that you will get while juicing will help improve the health and appearance of your skin and hair as well.

Benefit #8 – Give Your Immune System a Boost

Since so many people today do not get the fruits and vegetables that their body needs, it is no wonder that so many people have weakened immune systems. When you begin juicing on a regular basis, you will enjoy the benefit of giving your immune system a great boost. If you get colds or other illnesses on a regular basis, juicing may be just the thing to help you feel a lot better.

When you begin juicing regularly, you will start getting a wide variety of different antioxidants, which are needed to keep your immune system functioning the way it should. Some of the important antioxidants you will get from veggies and fruits include vitamin E, vitamin A and vitamin C. Phytochemicals are also found in many fruits and vegetables and they come with a variety of great health benefits, giving your immune system and your overall health a good boost.

Benefit #9 – Prevent Cancer

One of the more famous benefits of juicing is the benefit of cancer prevention. Since juicing gives you a wide variety of vitamins, minerals and antioxidants that your body needs, it arms your body to fight off cancer cells. When you juice on a regular basis and ensure you are getting all those important nutrients, you will be going a long way towards reducing your risk of getting cancer in the future.

Interestingly enough, juicing is often recommended to individuals who already have cancer. While it does not miraculously cure cancer right away, the antioxidants help to fight off cancer cells and give the immune system a boost so the body can work to fight off cancer on its own. When used along with other treatments, it can be an excellent method of beating cancer. Of course, if you are being treated for cancer, it is always important to follow the advice of your doctors and make sure you talk to them about juicing to ensure you avoid doing anything that may interfere with other treatments you may be given for cancer.

Benefit #10 – Slow the Aging Process

Last, juicing for weight loss can actually have the benefit of slowing down the aging process. Instead of wasting your money on all those expensive anti-aging creams and lotions, nature can offer you a great anti-aging treatment – fruits and veggies. Drinking fresh juices on a regular basis can provide your body with the nutrients it needs to stay young. Since free radicals are known to cause aging, getting plenty of antioxidants from the juice you drink will help to fight off free radicals, slowing down the aging process. People that get plenty of fruits and vegetables on a regular basis are often able to look younger and they are less likely to deal with health problems that come with aging as well.

Of course, these are only a few of the great benefits you can enjoy when you begin juicing. Juicing may also help to improve heart health, since you are less likely to eat foods that may lead to high blood pressure, high cholesterol and heart disease in the future. Juicing can also help you to lose weight, which is one of the more popular benefits individuals want to experience when they go on a juicing diet. As you begin juicing, you will fill up on low calorie fruits and vegetables in juice form, which will keep you from indulging in other unhealthy foods. Juicing also helps to cleanse out your body, eliminating toxins and waste, which can help you to lose weight as well. Just a few of the other benefits of juicing may include reducing problems with depression, strengthening your bones, improving eye health, rebuilding blood cells, keeping your body pH less acidic and reducing your risk of many different diseases.

Chapter 3: Helpful Tips to Simplify Juicing for Weight Loss

When you begin juicing for weight loss, you want to make sure that you get the best results from your juicing diet. The good news is that there are some great tips out there that can make juicing simpler and tips that can help you ensure you get the best nutrition when you make and drink these juices. To get the tastiest juices and the most benefits from juicing, the following are some top tips to keep in mind as you begin juicing and using the recipes you will find in this book.

Tip #1 – Choose Organic Fruits and Veggies if Possible

One of the best tips to remember when you begin juicing is to choose organic fruits and veggies if possible. Going with organic fruits and veggies helps you avoid pesticides, which you do not want to take in when trying to get all the goodness you can from juicing. Of course, certain fruits and veggies are worse than others when it comes to pesticides. The following fruits and veggies may have thinner skins, which make them more vulnerable to pesticides, so it is better to choose organically grown versions of these items:

- Kale
- Carrots
- Blueberries
- Spinach
- Lettuces
- Cucumbers
- Blueberries
- Strawberries
- Celery
- Collard Greens

If the fruit or vegetable has a thin skin, it is a good idea to choose the organic version of the fruit or veggie when you plan to use them for juicing.

Tip #2 – Learn About Great Additions that Make Juices Taste Better

When you first start juicing, you may find that some of the juices do not taste very good to you, especially those that only have vegetables in them. While you will get used to the taste over time, you can add some simple additions to juices to make them taste better to you. Here are a few of the best additions to add to juices when you need something to make them more palatable for you.

- **Cranberries** – If you like the flavor of cranberries, they can be added to juices to make them taste a bit better. They work well in green juices, since the cranberry flavor usually overpowers the greens. Not only will the cranberries add great flavor, but they offer a huge amount of antioxidants and phytonutrients as well.
- **Coconut** – Unsweetened shredded coconut or fresh coconut can be used to offer some flavor to juices as well. Coconut water can also be added to juices to add flavor and dilute them just a bit. Coconut has healthy fats in it, so it tastes good and offers great health benefits too.
- **Fresh Ginger** – You may notice that many of the juice recipes included in this juicing guide include fresh ginger. This is because ginger adds some great flavor, especially to vegetable juices that may not taste as good. Ginger also works to reduce bad cholesterol levels and offers great cardiovascular health benefits as well.
- **Limes and Lemons** – Limes and lemons have powerful flavors, which makes them the perfect addition to juices when you want to make them taste a little more palatable. Simple add in half of a lime or a lemon to any juice to improve the flavor. Just make sure you peel the lime or lemon and remove the seeds.

Tip #3 – Always Drink Juices as Soon as You Can Once You Juice Fruits and Veggies

One of the most important tips you can follow as you start juicing is to always drink juices as soon as you can one you have juiced the fruits and veggies. As time goes by, the juice will begin to lose some of its nutritional value. Sometimes the juice will turn a strange color as it begins to oxidize as well, although this does not mean that the juice has gone bad. It is best to drink the juice immediately. If you cannot drink the juice immediately, work to make sure you drink the juice within 24 hours for the best nutrition and taste. Fresh juices do not have any preservatives in them, so they can quickly go bad.

Tip #4 – Try Prepping Produce in Advance for Faster Juicing

Many people avoid juicing because they think that juicing will require a lot of work and time. Juicing actually can take quite a bit of your time, since you have to wash and cut up veggies and fruits before you can juice many of them. Since it can be easy to go off your juicing diet because it all feels like too much work, you may want to try prepping your produce in advance for faster juicing. Try preparing produce by washing it and cutting it up. You can do this a couple times a week so ingredients for juices are readily available. Simple place prepared produce in storage containers or plastic bags, then put them in the refrigerator. Then you can quickly get the ingredients out of the refrigerator and use them when needed. Of course, remember that veggies and fruits can start losing nutrients after you cut them, so if you prep ahead of time, avoid prepping veggies and fruits too far in advance so you avoid losing those important nutrients that your body needs.

Tip #5 – Clean Your Juicer Right Away and Clean Thoroughly

It is important that you clean your juicer right away, making sure that you clean it thoroughly. It is easy to put off cleaning the juicer because you are in a hurry, but this can quickly lead to big problems. If you do not quickly clean out the juice and pulp, it will begin to get sticky. This will make it even more difficult for you to get your juicer clean. If you have a high quality juicer, it should only take a few minutes to clean it when you are done juicing, which will save you a lot of time later on. If your juicer has a metal grater, one of the best tips for cleaning it is to keep a toothbrush around to get it clean.

Tip #6 – If You Do Store Juice, Store Carefully

While it is best to drink your juices quickly, you can store them. However, if you are going to store juices, make sure you store them carefully. Juices are best right away, but you can keep them stored for about 24 hours without too much of a problem. For the best results, make sure you place juice in a glass jar – avoid putting juice in a plastic container. Make sure that the jar has a lid that is airtight and fill the jar with juice right up to the top so you avoid having too much oxygen in the jar, which can damage your juice. Once you have the juice in the jar, make sure it is put in your refrigerator and keep it there until you are ready to drink the juice.

Tip #7 – Always Take the Time to Wash Produce

Always make sure you take the time to wash your produce thoroughly before you juice it. Fruit and vegetables may have contaminants on the outside, which you need to wash away to avoid contaminating your fruit. Even if you are going to remove the peeling or the rind, you still need to wash the produce well. Contamination can still occur if the skin or rind is removed.

Tip #8 – Avoid Peeling Fruits and Veggies that Can Be Eaten with the Skin

If you can eat the fruit or vegetable with the skin on, leave the skin on when you juice them. Many fruits and vegetables contain a large amount of nutrients within their skins, so removing the skins means that you are losing out on some great nutrition. For example, you can leave the skin on cucumbers, apples and even carrots when you are ready to juice them. Just make sure you wash them very well before juicing. Pay attention to the recipes within this juicing guide, since they will tell you when it is okay to leave the skin on the fruits or vegetables that go in the juice.

Tip #9 – Do Not Ruin Your Juice by Adding Sugar – There are Better Ways to Sweeten Juices

When you go on a juicing diet to lose weight, you are working to get away from sugar and processed foods. Do not ruin your juice by adding sugar to the juice if you think it needs a little sweetness. The great news is that there are many better ways that you can sweeten the juices a bit if you think they need it. For example, instead of sugar, a sugar alternative like Stevia, which happens to be all natural, can add some sweetness to the juice. A touch of honey can add some sweetness in a natural way as well. In many cases, just adding a sweet fruit to the juice can help you ensure that you get plenty of sweet flavor in the juice. There is never a need to add any sugar to these juice recipes.

Chapter 4: Delicious Juicing Recipes for Any Meal

If you're following the a juicing diet, you'll find that you can use juicing recipes for any meal or snack during the day. Juicing for weight loss can be extremely effective, but you want to ensure you have a wide variety of juices to enjoy so you don't get bored. The following are some wonderful recipes. Some include fruits, others are primarily made up of veggies and some even include both fruits and vegetables. You're sure to find some great juicing recipes that will tempt your taste buds while helping you lose some weight.

Orange Mango Juice Recipe

This juice combines together the delicious flavors of oranges and mangos. The addition of some kale leaves provides an extra nutritional punch when you consume this juice. You'll be able to make this juice very quickly and it's an especially tasty treat when you first get up in the morning. Add a little ice to make it extra cold and refreshing.

What You'll Need:

1 large mango
4 medium oranges
3-4 leaves of kale

How to Make It:

Wash the mango before using. Remove the skin from the mango, since some individuals may have a bad reaction to some of the chemicals naturally found in the mango's skin. Cut the pit of the mango out, then cut the mango into medium sized chunks.

Peel all four oranges. Break the oranges into 4-5 big sections that can easily be fed into the juice.

Was the kale leaves and shake them dry or dry with a paper towel.

Place mango chunks, orange sections and kale leave in a juice. Juice ingredients. Makes 1-2 servings. Drink immediately for the best taste.

Refreshing Red Pepper and Basil Juice Recipe

Along with refreshing, tasty red bell pepper, this juice is packed with great veggies. It includes cucumbers, broccoli, carrot, celery and chia seeds, which pack in plenty of great nutrients. The basil really gives the flavor a boost, as does the lime. The tabasco adds a kick, but you can eliminate the tabasco if you don't like it.

What You'll Need:

1 large bunch of broccoli
1 handful of fresh basil leaves
1 carrot, small
1 small cucumber
1 red bell pepper, large
½ lime, with the rind
2 teaspoons of chia seeds
2 celery stalks
½ cup of Jicama with the skin
Tabasco sauce to taste (optional)

How to Make It:

Wash broccoli, basil leaves, carrot, cucumber, red bell pepper, celery and Jicama.

Remove pepper top, seeds and innards from the red bell pepper. Cut broccoli into chunks. Peel carrot and cut carrot into chunks. Leave peeling on cucumber but cut cucumber into chunks that will fit into your juicer. Chop celery into chunks as well.

Place broccoli, basil leaves, carrot, cucumber, bell pepper, lime, celery stalks and Jicama into the juicer. Juice until finished. Place juice in a bottle or pitcher. Add tabasco if desired and chia seeds. Mix well. Serve immediately.

Lime Spinach Juice Recipe

All the spinach in this juice offers many great nutrients your body needs, such as potassium and iron. The baby carrots add even more vitamins and minerals that are important. The lime and green apple added to the juice provide a delicious flavor that will make you wish you doubled this recipe.

What You'll Need:

1 medium green apple
1 large cucumber
5-6 baby carrots
2 large handfuls of spinach
1 lime

How to Make It:

Wash the green apple, cutting it into chunks, leaving skin on the apple. Wash cucumber and leave it's skin on too, cutting into chunks. Wash spinach carefully, allowing to drain in a colander. Wash lime, remove the skin and then cut up the lime into chunks.

Add apple chunks, cucumber chunks, carrots, spinach and lime chunks into the juicer. Juice the ingredients.

Serve juice right away.

NOTE: If you like your juice a bit sweeter, simply add another apple to the juice for some extra sweetness.

Wild Edible Greens Juice Recipe

If you have a lot of wild, edible greens around your home, these fresh greens can be added to your juice for a healthy, delicious juice. Just make sure you know which greens are edible, since you want to avoid eating anything that could be dangerous. Have fun finding out about fresh wild greens. You can look online or even buy a book that will help you to identify greens that you can eat.

What You'll Need:

½ cucumber
1 large lemon
1 ½ pounds of fresh wild greens (such as sow thistle, chick weed, yellow dock, dandelion or miner's lettuce)
1 inch piece of fresh ginger root
3-4 bok choy stalks
6 celery tops

How to Make It:

Start by washing all the fresh wile greens you have collected, allowing them to drain in a colander before using them in the juice. Wash cucumber, lemon, bok choy and celery tops as well. Leave the skin on the cucumber, cutting it up into pieces that will easily fit in your juicer. Chop bok choy stalks into smaller pieces and cut up celery tops if needed.

Add all ingredients to the juicer, juicing until complete. Makes about 24 ounces of wild edible greens juice, which is about two servings. Drink the juice immediately.

Tasty Morning Apple and Carrot Juice Recipe

This delicious juice is a wonderful juice to make in the morning for a great pick me up. It's tasty and packed with great nutrients to help fuel you through the day. The beet adds some great vitamins and minerals, but you won't taste it with the green apples in the juice, offering a nice sweet and tart flavor.

What You'll Need:

1/2 beet
2 medium green apples
1 stalk of celery with leaves
2 medium sized carrots

How to Make It:

Wash the apples, celery and carrots. Cut a beet in half, peeling carefully and cutting into chunks. Leave the peeling on the apples, but core the apple and then cut it into pieces. The celery should be cut up as well. Peel carrots, cutting into large pieces.

Place the beet, apples, celery and carrots into a juicer and then process. Serve the juice up right away for a great way to start the morning.

Carrot Citrus Twist Juice Recipe

The carrots in this delicious juice recipe pack great nutrients, offering one of the best ways to get vitamin A. Some of the other important minerals carrots provide include copper, potassium, calcium and iron. While carrot juice tastes great by itself, adding the citrus to the recipe really gives it a tangy, sweet twist. Not only do the oranges add great flavor, but they add a huge amount of vitamin C to your juice as well. Try this delicious juice recipe over ice. It makes a great juice to drink for breakfast.

What You'll Need:

2 large oranges, peeled and seeded
8 large carrots, unpeeled

How to Make It:

Start by peeling the oranges, making sure you remove any seeds. Break up the oranges into large sections so they will fit into your juicer.

Wash the carrots well, removing any dirt. However, leave the skin on the carrots, since the skin is packed with great nutrients. Cut the tops off the carrots. Cut carrots into chunks.

Place oranges and carrots into the juicer, juicing. Makes 2 glasses of juice.

Tangy Grapefruit Carrot Juice Recipe

With eight carrots in this recipe, you'll get a large dose of vitamin A and other essential vitamins and minerals your body needs. You get a tangy surprise to this juice by adding the grapefruit. Grapefruits also pack in plenty of great nutrients, such as vitamin C. Some studies even show that grapefruit can even help you boost your weight loss efforts. While the mint is optional in this juice recipe, it really adds to the flavor. Mint also helps to reduce stomach problems and may help prevent cancer as well.

What You'll Need:

2 medium grapefruits
8 unpeeled large carrots
1 mint sprig, fresh (optional)

How to Make It:

Get started by washing the grapefruits, then peeling it and removing any seeds. Break the grapefruits into large sections to make them easily fit into your juicer. Wash the carrots well, but leave the peels on. Take the tops off the carrots as well. Take time to wash the mint before using.

Start by juicing the mint, then run the grapefruit and carrots through the juicer, which should bring out the any mint juice left in the juicer. Serve the juice immediately.

For a nice, refreshing twist, add the juice to a blender, adding in some ice. Blend until you have a slushy mixture. This cold, delicious twist to the juice recipe is wonderful on a very hot day.

Very Veggie Blast Juice Recipe

This juice recipe is packed with many great veggies, including carrots, celery, kale, radishes, tomatoes, bell peppers and more. The apple that is added to the mix adds some sweetness and the fresh ginger root gives the juice a nice kick. You'll get a wide ranges of vitamins and minerals when you whip up this delicious juice recipe.

What You'll Need:

1 red bell pepper
3 celery stalks
1 medium tomato
1 beet
2 inches of turmeric root
½ bunch of kale
2-3 inch chunk of Daikon radish
1 large carrot
3-4 leaves of basil
½ bunch of fresh cilantro
1 green apple
1 inch of fresh ginger root

How to Make It:

Begin by washing the bell pepper, celery stalks, tomato,

beet, kale, radish, carrot, basil leaves, cilantro and apple. Remove seeds and top from the pepper, cutting pepper into large chunks. Chop celery stalks into chunks. Cut the tomato into quarters. Cut the beet into quarters or smaller to make it fit through your juicer. Remove the top of the carrot, but leave peeling on the carrot. Core the green apple and cut into chunks.

Process all the ingredients through a juicer. When juicing is complete, take the leftover pulp and process it in the juicer again. Serve juice right away and avoid saving leftovers.

Bone Building Kale Juice Recipe

Keeping your bones healthy and strong is important, and this juice recipe is packed with great ingredients that include vitamins and minerals that will help keep bones healthy. The kale included in the juice includes vitamin K, vitamin A, vitamin C, iron, calcium and beta carotene. The carrots offer more beta carotene and vitamin A. The apple adds some fiber and sweetness to the juice and even the parsley offers many great health benefits as well.

What You'll Need:

5 large kale leaves
1 medium green apple
5 large carrots
4-6 sprigs of parsley

How to Make It:

Wash the kale leaves and the parsley sprigs and allow them to drain in a colander. Wash the carrots well, removing any dirt. Cut the tops off the carrots but leave the peelings on them. Wash the apple, then core the apple. Leave the apple skin in place, since it includes great nutrients.

Process the kale leaves, green apple, carrots and parsley in the juicer. Cut ingredients into chunks if needed to fit through the juicer. After ingredients are juiced, drink the juice immediately for the best taste and nutritional punch.

*NOTE: a masticating juicer works best for this recipe and others that include leafy greens

Iron Packed Spinach Broccoli Juice Recipe

Getting plenty of iron in your diet is important, since iron helps with the production of red blood cells and the transportation of oxygen throughout your body. If you are not getting enough iron, you could experience symptoms that include headaches, low energy, weak hair and fingernails, shortness of breath and rapid heartbeat. This juice is made with iron packed veggies that help you get a great dose of iron when you drink this juice. Drinking it on a regular basis can help improve your iron levels and the ingredients also provide other important nutrients your body needs as well.

What You'll Need:

2 stalks of broccoli
2 beetroots
8-10 large spinach leaves

How to Make It:

Start by washing the beetroots and the broccoli stalks. Wash the spinach leaves and allow them to drain before juicing. Cut the beetroots and broccoli stalks into large pieces that will go through your juicer.

Juice the ingredients. Enjoy this juice immediately for the best benefits. Makes about 2 servings.

Citrus and Cabbage Juice Recipe

This delicious juice recipe includes a variety of different vegetables and fruits, which means you'll get plenty of nutrients when you drink it. It makes a great juice to start out your day with. The spinach and beetroot offer plenty of iron and the citrus offers a great supply of vitamin C, which helps your body better use the iron. The cabbage included in the juice provides many health benefits as well, including slowing down the aging process and helping to prevent certain types of cancer. All the citrus fruits included in this recipe means you will get a sweet, tangy flavor and you probably will not taste the cabbage and other veggies at all.

What You'll Need:

¼ head of cabbage
5-6 leaves of spinach
1 kiwifruit
½ a large grapefruit
½ of a medium beetroot
1 stalk of broccoli
1 large orange
½ of a large lemon
1 inch piece of fresh ginger

How to Make It:

Wash the cabbage and spinach leaves, allowing them to drain in a colander before juicing. Peel the kiwifruit, grapefruit, orange and lemon. Make sure that you remove any seeds in the grapefruit, orange and lemon. Was the beetroot and broccoli.

Begin by juicing the cabbage, spinach and broccoli. Once they are done juicing, add the ginger and the citrus fruits. When complete, make sure everything is mixed together well. This makes enough juice for at least two servings, so enjoy sharing this juice with a friend or family member instead of saving it.

Cucumber and Tomato Immune Boosting Juice Recipe

Juicing not only provides a great way to lose some weight, but it also can help you boost your immune system as well. This juice in particular is filled with ingredients that will give your immune system a nice boost. The parsley has high iron content and is a great antioxidant that helps to fight off bacteria. The garlic has antibacterial and antiseptic properties, which can boost your immune system as well. Lycopene comes from the tomatoes in the juice, which can help prevent certain types of cancer. While this is not a sweet juice, it has a nice, wholesome, savory taste that you are sure to enjoy.

What You'll Need:

1 large handful of fresh parsley
½ cucumber, unpeeled
2 large tomatoes
1 clove of garlic, peeled
2 stalks of celery
1/8 of a medium sized onion (try a sweet onion like a Vidalia for better flavor)

How to Make It:

Wash the parsley carefully and allow to drain. Wash the cucumber and leave the peeling on, since it includes important nutrients. Wash tomatoes, cutting into large chunks. Peel the garlic clove. Wash celery and onion. Cut celery into chunks.

Add the parsley to the juicer first, since parsley does not provide a whole lot of juice. After juicing the parsley, juice the cucumber, tomatoes, garlic, celery and onion. Pour the mixture into a glass, making sure it is well mixed up. Drink immediate for the best results. Makes a single serving of juice.

Sweet Pineapple Watermelon Juice Recipe

Watermelon is such a sweet, refreshing fruit, especially on a hot day. It is high in vitamin B6, which is known to help reduce tension. If you have a tough day ahead, this juice a great choice. The lemon and pineapple add even more nutrients that are important and plenty of delicious flavor as well. With all the sweetness of this juice, you may want to serve it up over ice for a cool, sweet treat that is actually good for you.

What You'll Need:

¼ of a watermelon
½ of a pineapple
½ of a lemon

How to Make It:

Remove the rind from the watermelon. If the watermelon has seeds, make sure that you remove them before you begin juicing. Remove the rind from the pineapple and peel the lemon. Remove any seeds from the lemon as well. Cut the watermelon and the pineapple into manageable chunks so they are easier for you to juice.

Juice the watermelon, pineapple and lemon. Once you are done juicing, mix the juice well to ensure it is well combined. Drink right away. Serve it over some ice or add it to the blender with a cup or so of ice and blend for a frosty, delicious drink.

Kiwi Strawberry Energy Boosting Juice Recipe

If you need a great boost of energy, try this delicious kiwi strawberry energy boosting juice recipe. It can be a great way to start your day or you can make this juice to drink before you work out. This way you have plenty of energy to help you make the most of your exercise routine. The kiwi, apple, strawberries and lime all give this juice a sweet taste. If you want to make it a little sweeter, you can also mix in just a bit of organic Stevia to the juice before you drink it.

What You'll Need:

½ of a lime
6 large strawberries
4 large kale leaves
2 kiwis, peeled
2 medium green apples
Pinch of organic Stevia (optional)

How to Make It:

Peel the lime and remove and seeds. Wash strawberries, removing the tops. Wash the kale leaves and allow to drain. Wash and peel the kiwis. Wash and then core the apples, leaving on the peels.

Juice the lime, strawberries, kale leaves, kiwis and green apples. Pour into a glass and enjoy this sweet drink right away. Enjoy the natural rush of energy.

Citrus, Apple, Pear Juice Recipe

Pears are a sweet, delicious fruit that happens to be rich in vitamin K, vitamin C and vitamin A. This fruit is also known to help improve digestion, which is important for cleansing out the body. Combined with the tartness of green apples and delicious citrus fruits, this juice will make your taste buds sing. Have fun trying the recipes with several different types of pears, such as red Anjou pears, Bosc pears or the wonderful Asian pears.

What You'll Need:

2 medium pears (choose the pear of your choice)
2 large carrots
1 large orange
1 medium tangerine
1 large granny smith apple

How to Make It:

Wash the pears, removing the core and seeds; however, the peeling can be left on the pears. The carrots should be washed and topped, leaving the peels. Peel the orange and tangerine after washing them, breaking into large sections. Wash and then core the granny smith apple, leaving the peel on the apple as well.

Run the pears, carrots, orange, tangerine and apple through the juicer. Pour the juice over ice and drink it right away. If the juice is too thick or strong, you can always add a bit of water to get the juice to your desired consistency and taste.

Beta Carotene Deluxe Juice Recipe

You are guaranteed to get a huge dose of beta carotene when you drink this delicious juice. It includes delicious cantaloupe, which is known to include many different vitamins and minerals essential to your body. Vitamin C and vitamin A are just a few of the important vitamins included in cantaloupe. You will also find that it includes a high concentration of potassium as well.

What You'll Need:

1 medium cantaloupe
4 medium sized carrots
1 large sweet potato

How to Make It:

Wash the cantaloupe and then remove the rind. However, you should try to leave a bit of the greenish rind behind to juice, since it offers many great nutrients. Wash the carrots and top them, leaving the peelings. Wash the sweet potato thoroughly, leaving the peel on the sweet potato as well.

Juice the cantaloupe, carrots and sweet potato. Make sure the juice is well mixed to combine the flavors. Drink immediate for a large amount of beta carotene.

Antioxidant Mixed Berry Juice Recipe

When it comes to getting antioxidants, berries happen to have more antioxidants than most other fruits. Antioxidants found in the berries help to protect the body against damage from free radicals. Many berries can also aid in weight loss, since raspberries are known to include ketones that help burn off fat and strawberries can help keep blood sugar levels stable. Strawberries include more than 100% of the daily value of vitamin C and other berries like blackberries and blueberries include a high amount of vitamin C as well. The addition of mango to this juice recipe adds even more vitamin C and a nice dose of vitamin A as well. The apples add some great fiber, which will fill you up and help keep your digestive system working the way it should. This juice will taste wonderful when blended with some ice or simply served over ice, offering a chilly, refreshing, healthy drink that will taste great at any time of day.

What You'll Need:

1 cup of blueberries
1 cup of strawberries
½ cup of raspberries
½ cup of blackberries

½ cup of cubed mango

1 green apple

How to Make It:

Wash the blueberries, strawberries, raspberries and blackberries. Remove the stems from the strawberries. Wash a mango and peel it, cubing up a ½ cup of the mango. Save the rest of the mango for another juicing recipe. Wash the apple and then core it and remove its seeds. Leave the apple peeling in place.

Pass the blueberries, strawberries, raspberries, blackberries, mango and apple through a juicer. Juice the apple last, since it will help clean out some of the berry juices left behind. Pour over ice or mix in a blender with a cup of ice. Drink immediately for a nice dose of antioxidants.

Coconut Mango Tropical Delight Juice Recipe

Mangos have a delicious, sweet flavor. Not only do they taste great, but they include high amounts of vitamin C and pectin as well, which can help lower blood pressure and cholesterol. The vitamin A included in mangos can help keep eyes healthy as well. The one problem people often have with mangos is figuring out if they are ripe or not. A ripe mango should have a bit of give to the outside skin and should have a nice, sweet scent as well. The addition of coconut water and several tropical fruits makes this juice recipe a delight for your taste buds.

What You'll Need:

1 large mango, prepared
2 medium oranges
2 cups of pineapple, cubed
1 lime
½ inch piece of fresh ginger
Coconut water, to your own taste

How to Make It:

To prepare the mango for juicing, start by washing the skin carefully to ensure the flesh is not contaminated. The pit must be removed from the mango, which can be done by slicing around the pit and pulling sections apart to pop out the pit. Use a sharp knife to score the mango flesh, then scooping out the flesh with a spoon, ensuring the rind is left behind.

Wash and peel the oranges and ensure pineapple is cubed small enough to easily go through the juicer. Peel the lime and remove any seeds. Wash ginger before juicing as well.

Run the mango flesh, oranges, pineapple, lime and ginger through the juicer. Mix the finished juice with some coconut water until you have the flavor you prefer. Drink at room temperature or pour over ice for a refreshing tropical treat.

Pear, Apple, Blueberry Juice Recipe

Blueberries are not just wonderfully juicy and sweet, but these small berries include a high amount of antioxidants as well. This fruit is known to help reduce the risk of inflammation and may help protect against certain types of cancer as well. Since these berries have such thin skin, it is a good idea to use organic berries whenever possible. This juice recipe adds the delicate flavor of pears and the sweet, tartness of granny smith apples as well, making a juice that is packed with flavor and great nutrients for the body. Enjoy changing up the flavor a bit by using different kinds of pears in the juice.

What You'll Need:

1 cup of blueberries
½ cup of strawberries
½ cup of blackberries
1 pear, any kind
2 granny smith apples

How to Make It:

Wash the blueberries, strawberries and blackberries. Remove the tops from the strawberries. Wash the pear and the apple. Remove the core and stem from the pear, cutting the pear into large chunks. Core the apple, leave the skin on and then cut the apple into large pieces.

Run the blueberries, strawberries and blackberries through the juicer first. Then, run the pear and apples through the juicer, cleaning out the berry juices when they go through the juicer. Fill a glass with ice cubes and pour juice over the ice. Drink the juice right away to get the most nutrients from the ingredients.

Carrot and Cucumber Broccoli Juice Recipe

The broccoli included in this juice is high in both vitamin C and vitamin E, which are known to help support the immune system. This vegetable also has anti-carcinogenic properties and some evidence shows that broccoli may help prevent cancer. Although broccoli offers great nutrition, it is low in calories, which means it is a great addition to your juices if you are trying to lose weight. When juicing the broccoli, make sure you juice the head and the stalks for the nutrition. The carrots and cucumbers add more flavor and nutrition to this juice.

What You'll Need:

1 large cucumber
3 stalks of celery, including the leaves
1 stalk of broccoli, including the head and the stalk
3 large carrots

How to Make It:

Begin by washing the cucumber, celery and carrots. Clean the broccoli very well, since the head often traps bacteria and dirt. Leave the peeling on the cucumber and cut into large chunks. Cut the celery into chunks as well. Do not peel the carrots, but make sure you remove the tops, then cutting the carrots into large pieces. Cut the broccoli into small enough pieces to easily fit into your juicer.

Run the cucumber, celery, broccoli and carrots through your juicer. When done juicing, serve up the juice right away. This juice is usually best at room temperature.

Delicious Tropical Papaya and Pineapple Juice Recipe

Since pineapple has such a high water content, it is a great fruit to use when juicing, providing plenty of juice. Pineapple is high in minerals like manganese and vitamins, such as vitamin C. The sweetness of the pineapple is delicious with other fruits that are more tart. To get the most out of your pineapple when juicing, add the core of the pineapple to the juicer as well, since it offers a lot of bromelain. The other tropical fruits in this juice, such as the papaya, guava and mango, really add a complexity of flavors to this juice.

What You'll Need:

1 large orange, peeled
1 cup of papaya, cubed
1 cup of pineapple, cubed
1 guava
½ of a large mango

How to Make It:

Rinse off the orange and then peel it, removing any seeds. Break the orange up into large sections. Prepare a papaya and cube up a cup of it for the juice. Cube up a cup of pineapple, including some of the core. Prepare the guava for juicing. Wash the mango, removing the pit and using half of the mango flesh for this recipe. Save the rest of the mango for another juice recipe.

Run the orange, papaya, pineapple, guava and mango through the juicer. Fill a large glass with crushed ice, pouring the juice over the ice. Serve the juice immediately for the best flavor and nutrition. This juice is so delicious that you may want to double the recipe and share some with a friend.

Pineapple and Kale Detoxifying Juice Recipe

This recipe includes all the benefits of pineapple, including bromelain, vitamin C and manganese. It also includes great nutrition from the kale included, as well as wonderful nutrients from the cucumber, lemon and mint. This juice is a great detoxifying recipe. For the best results, make this recipe and drink the juice throughout an entire day. Refrigerate the juice until needed but make sure all the juice is consumed within 24 hours or less.

What You'll Need:

2 large cucumbers, unpeeled
½ of a lemon, peeled and seeded
½ cup of pineapple, including the core
1 large bunch of mint
1 large bunch of kale, stems removed
¼ inch of fresh ginger

How to Make It:

Rinse the cucumber thoroughly, leaving the peelings in place. Chunk the cucumbers into large pieces. Wash the lemon, peel it and then remove any seeds. Prepare the pineapple, ensuring it is cubed and include a bit of the core with the pineapple chunks. Wash the mint leaves and kale in a colander, allowing to drain thoroughly before juicing. Wash the ginger as well.

Process the cucumbers, lemon, pineapple, mint, kale and ginger in the juicer. Place the juice in a pitcher. Drink one cup of the juice right away. Store leftovers in the refrigerator and consume throughout the day. Ensure all the juice is consumed within one day for the best results.

Fruity Cleansing Juice Recipe

Many people choose to go on the juicing diet to cleanse their body and lose weight. While there are many delicious juicing recipes that can be used to accomplish these goals, this fruity cleansing recipe is a delicious, nutritious way to begin cleansing the body. All the fruits included provide plenty of vitamins and minerals, not to mention you are sure to appreciate the delicious, fruity flavor as well.

What You'll Need:

1 granny smith apple
½ cup of blueberries
½ cup of raspberries
2 large peaches
2 large oranges, peeled

How to Make It:

To begin making the fruity cleansing juice recipe, start by washing the granny smith apple, the blueberries, raspberries, peaches and oranges. After all the fruits have been washed, remove the core and seeds from the apple, leaving the peeling intact. Remove the seeds from the peaches, but leave the peach skins intact. Peel the oranges, removing any seeds. Cut the apple and peaches into large pieces and break the oranges into large sections.

Process the blueberries, raspberries, peaches and oranges in a juicer. Run the apple pieces through the juicer last. Drink the juice right away. For the best cleansing results, drink the juice while it is at room temperature.

Go Green Spinach and Cucumber Juice Recipe

This delicious juice recipe is all about the greens. It has cucumbers, parsley, spinach, celery and even a granny smith apple in it. All the spinach offers a great dose of potassium and iron. Not only does this juice provide many essential vitamins and minerals that your body needs, but also the juice is also great for detoxifying your body. If you do not like the flavor, you can always add a second apple to the recipe to add some extra sweetness.

What You'll Need:

2 large handfuls of baby spinach
1 stalk of celery, with the leaves
1 large cucumber
1 large handful of fresh parsley
1 large granny smith apple

How to Make It:

Use a colander and rinse the baby spinach and parsley, allowing the leaves to drain in the colander until they are well drained. Wash the celery, cucumber and the apple. Chop the celery into large pieces. Leave the peeling on the cucumber and chop it into large chunks.

Core the apple, making sure all seeds are removed. Do not remove the peel. Cut the apple into pieces.

Run the spinach and parsley through the juicer first, since they do not provide as much juice. Then, run the celery, cucumber and apple through the juicer last. Blend together all the juices. Serve this juice over some ice in a tall glass. Enjoy immediately.

Spinach and Cinnamon Metabolism Booster Juice Recipe

If you are juicing for weight loss, you want to consume juices that will give your metabolism a nice boost. After all, if you have been eating processed foods for many years, your metabolism may have slowed down, which can make it more difficult for you to lose weight. This recipe will help give your metabolism a nice boost and it is packed with ingredients that help to blast away fat as well. The cinnamon adds a nice touch to the juice and is known to help stabilize blood sugar levels.

What You'll Need:

1 cup of spinach leaves
4 large carrots, unpeeled
1 lemon
1 stalk of celery with the leaves
¼ teaspoon of cinnamon
1 granny smith green apple

How to Make It:

Start out by placing the spinach leaves in a colander, rinsing them very well before using. Allow to drain a bit before juicing them. Wash the carrots, topping them but leaving the peelings on them. The lemon should be peeled and the seeds removed after washing it. Wash the celery and apple as well. Cut the celery into big pieces. Core the apple and then cut into pieces too.

Run the spinach leaves from the juicer first. Then run the carrots, celery, lemon and apple through your juicer. After juicing, mix the cinnamon into the juice, stirring well to combine. If the lemon makes the juice a bit tart, use a bit of purified water to dilute it a bit before drinking. Drink right away and enjoy the boost to your metabolism.

Green Juice with a Hint of Sweetness Recipe

This is a green juice recipe that includes all green ingredients. While it includes greens like kale, romaine and parsley, the apple adds a touch of sweetness to the juice. With all the greens in the juice, this is a drink that is packed with vitamins and minerals that will fuel your body and offer plenty of energy for your day. Try drinking this juice if you are feeling a bit tired or you feel like your immune system needs a boost.

What You'll Need:

3 stalks of celery

2 cups of fresh parsley

1 granny smith apple

2 cups of kale leaves

1 large cucumber

3 cups of romaine lettuce

How to Make It:

The celery, cucumber and apple should all be washed. The parsley, kale and romaine leaves can be washed in a colander and allowed to drain and dry a bit before you place them in a juicer.

Cut the celery and cucumber into chunks, leaving the peeling on the cucumber. Do not peel the apple, but core it and then cut into large apple chunks.

Process the parsley, kale leaves and romaine lettuce in the juicer first. Then run the celery, apple and cucumber through the juicer. Make sure you mix up the juicer very well to ensure you get the hint of sweetness throughout the entire batch of juice. Serve the juice immediately.

Potassium Delight Spinach Juice Recipe

Potassium is an important nutrient that your body needs. If you do not get enough potassium, you may suffer from muscle cramps and other symptoms. This juice can help you ensure that you are getting enough potassium in your diet, since the spinach is extremely high in potassium. The lemon juice adds some great flavor to the juice.

What You'll Need:

1 granny smith or other green apple
1 stalk of celery
1 handful of fresh baby spinach leaves
4 medium carrots, tops and greens removed
½ lemon
1 handful of fresh parsley

How to Make It:

Thoroughly rinse off the apple, celery, carrots and lemon. Use a colander to rinse the baby spinach leaves and parsley, letting the leaves dry some before using them in the juice. Without removing the peeling, core the apple and cut into quarters. Cut the celery into large pieces. Remove the carrot tops and chop carrots into big chunks. Peel the lemon and ensure any seeds have been removed before juicing.

Juice the parsley and the spinach leaves first. Place the apple, celery, lemon and carrots in the juicer. Juice. Ensure the juice is well mixed together for the best flavor. Serve the juice right away.

V-8 Flavored Juice Recipe

If you like the flavor of V-8 juice, this juice recipe is a great choice for you to try. You get the great flavor of the juice with even more vegetables and you can be sure of the ingredients going into the juice. With all the great vegetables in this juice, it has plenty of great flavor. The hot sauce really adds a nice pop to the juice, although it is optional and you do not have to add it if you do not like hot sauce. Whip this juice up on a hot day and enjoy the taste of vegetable goodness while getting all those important vitamins and other needed nutrients.

What You'll Need:

2 large tomatoes
2 medium carrots
2 teaspoons of lemon juice
¼ cup of water
1 large handful of spinach leaves
2 stalks of celery
2 cloves of garlic
¼ of a sweet Vidalia onion or other sweet onion
Hot sauce to taste (optional)

How to Make It:

Thoroughly wash the tomatoes, carrots, celery and onion. Rinse leaves well within a colander and let them drain. Peel the garlic cloves. Chop tomatoes into quarters or eights, making sure they will fit in the juicers. Chop the carrots, celery and onion into large chunks.

Place the spinach in the juicer and process. Add the tomatoes, carrots, celery, garlic and onion in the juicer and juice. Once the juice is complete, add the lemon juice and water. Mix together until well combined. Add the hot sauce to the juice to your own taste. Serve the juice right away and enjoy the nice combination of vegetable flavors.

Blueberry and Pomegranate Fruit Juice Recipe

Pomegranates are very high in antioxidants and vitamins, such as vitamin C. This fruit is known to help lower cholesterol and reduce the risk of heart disease. While pomegranates are delicious, preparing them for juicing can be a bit perplexing. Instead of eating the flesh of the pomegranate, the seeds of the fruit are actually eaten instead. This juice recipe not only includes pomegranates, but it includes blueberries and grapes as well, which add even more vitamins and antioxidants to this incredibly healthy and delicious juice. The wonderful sweetness makes it a great juice to enjoy when you want something sweet and refreshing.

What You'll Need:

1 cup of fresh organic blueberries
2 cups of red grapes
1 pomegranate, only the seeds

How to Make It:

To prepare the pomegranate, start by cutting the knob off the top of the fruit. Then use a very sharp knife to score the fruit, scoring in quarters. Pull away the sections of the rind. Hold the rind over cold water, popping the seeds off the rind. In the cold water, use your fingers to get the membranes off the seeds. Do this gently to avoid damaging the seeds. Simply allow the pith to go to the top of the water and remove it. Drain the seeds.

Wash the blueberries and the grapes thoroughly in a colander before you juice them, even if they are organic.

Place the pomegranate seeds in the juicer first, juicing them. Then process the blueberries and the red grapes, juicing them. Mix the juices together when complete. Pour the juice over some ice and enjoy right away.

Pumpkin Pineapple Juice Recipe

If you are making juices during the fall, you will definitely want to give this recipe a try, since pumpkins are more readily available during the fall months. Pumpkins offer excellent nutrition and they are very rich in vitamins like vitamin C and vitamin A. These vitamins can help to keep skin healthy, prevent aging and keep your immune system strong. The addition of pineapple and apples to this juice gives it a tropical flavor and the spices really give the juice a great taste.

What You'll Need:

½ cup of pineapple chunks
1 small pumpkin
2 green apples, such as granny smith
¼ teaspoon of allspice
¼ teaspoon of ginger
Purified water to taste

How to Make It:

Make sure the pumpkin is washed before you begin working with it. Then you will want cut the top off the pumpkin, scooping out the pumpkin flesh. Make sure you remove the seeds from the pumpkin flesh and do not put the pumpkin rind in the juicer.

Wash the apples and then core them to ensure all the seeds are removed. Leave the peelings on the apples.

Run the pumpkin flesh through the juicer. If you have a lot of pulp left, you can run it through the juicer again to extract more juice. Then, juice the pineapple and the apples. Mix the juices all together. Add the allspice and the ginger to the juice, mixing to combine. Add purified water to the juice until you have a flavor you enjoy. Drink the juice right away.

Body Cleansing Celery Juice Recipe

Celery is a great ingredient for cleaning out your body. It has a lot of water in it, which helps cleanse out the body. While this juice will help cleanse your body, it also contains some great nutrients from the spinach included. The beet included is a great cleansing ingredient as well. Drink this juice and enjoy getting a nice cleanse, which will help you lose weight and feel healthier. While the juice does have a very strong green taste to it, it really works so give it a try.

What You'll Need:

1 bunch of fresh cilantro
4 stalks of celery with the leaves
1 large handful of spinach
½ a beet

How to Make It:

Wash the beet and the celery stalks carefully. Cut the celery and the ½ a beet into pieces so they can be easily juiced. Place the cilantro and the spinach in a large colander, running water over them to rinse the leaves well. Allow to drain for a few minutes before you begin juicing.

Process the cilantro and the spinach through the juicer first. Last, add the celery and beet to the juicer, juicing until complete. Make sure that you mix the juices together very well to combined the flavors. Place in a glass and drink right away. If you are not fond of the flavor, try drinking it quickly while it is lukewarm to quickly get it down.

Chapter 5: Your 7 Day Juicing Diet Meal Plan

As you go on your juicing diet, you may be a bit unfamiliar with how to get started. To help you more easily begin the juicing diet, we've developed a helpful 7-day juicing diet meal plan to help you through those first days. Keep in mind, after a few days of juicing, you should go back to a regular diet. Juicing long term is usually unhealthy. However, even after you spend some time on the juicing diet, you can continue to use these recipes to replace a meal during your day as you continue to lead a healthy lifestyle. These juices are also great if your body is feeling a bit down and you want to get a large dose of great nutrients that your body needs. Begin your diet using this meal plan for great results. Feel free to mix and match days up if you want to keep things interesting and to your own unique taste.

Day 1:

Breakfast: Pineapple and Kale Detoxifying Juice Recipe

Lunch: Carrot and Cucumber Broccoli Juice Recipe

Dinner: Go Green Spinach and Cucumber Juice Recipe

Day 2:

Breakfast: Fruity Cleansing Juice Recipe

Lunch: Potassium Delight Spinach Juice Recipe

Dinner: Citrus and Cabbage Juice Recipe

Day 3:

Breakfast: Delicious Tropical Papaya and Pineapple Juice Recipe

Lunch: Iron Packed Spinach Broccoli Juice Recipe

Dinner: Green Juice with a Hint of Sweetness Recipe

Day 4:

Breakfast: Pear, Apple, Blueberry Juice Recipe

Lunch: Sweet Pineapple Watermelon Juice Recipe

Dinner: V-8 Flavored Juice Recipe

Day 5:

Breakfast: Coconut Mango Tropical Delight Juice Recipe

Lunch: Spinach and Cinnamon Metabolism Booster Juice Recipe

Dinner: Pumpkin Pineapple Juice Recipe

Day 6:

Breakfast: Blueberry and Pomegranate Fruit Juice Recipe

Lunch: Beta Carotene Deluxe Juice Recipe

Dinner: Cucumber and Tomato Immune Boosting Juice Recipe

Day 7:

Breakfast: Body Cleansing Celery Juice Recipe

Lunch: Antioxidant Mixed Berry Juice Recipe

Dinner: Citrus, Apple, Pear Juice Recipe

Section 2: Juicing Diet

Juicing diets have become a popular choice for just about anyone who wants to remove toxins from their body while enjoying fresh, natural foods. These cleansing beverages provide your body with plenty of liquid, keeping it hydrated and healthy. Because you can enjoy so many different kinds of juices, it's easy to stick to the plan without feeling excessively deprived or hungry. Many juice diets provide a small amount of weight loss, due to their inherently low-calorie nature.

This kind of diet plan has to be done correctly for optimum results, however. Simply replacing all your food with juice or going on a prolonged juice fast could deprive your body of essential nutrients, leaving you feeling more tired and unhealthy than you did when you began. That's why it's so important to drink a variety of juices throughout the day. This book will help you understand how to use juice to kick start a healthy lifestyle and keep yourself feeling healthy and energized through the power of juice. All the recipes are inspired by existing ones available on the Web, but they've been improved for this publication.

What Are Juicing Diets

It's important to understand what a juicing diet is and what it isn't. When used properly, juice diets last between three and 10 days and consist of carefully-chosen ingredients designed to keep your body operating correctly. They use only the freshest, best fruits and vegetables, including a variety of different juices every day. Ideally these foods are all made from organic produce that has been exposed to relatively few chemicals, in order to reduce the toxin load on your body.

While they can help you lose weight, juice diets aren't the right choice for large amounts of fat loss or long term use, since extreme use of juice fasting can actually cause damage to your systems. If you want to prepare your body for a healthy new routine and remove the toxins related to your old lifestyle, however, you can't go wrong with pure, natural juice.

The Benefits of Juicing

Juicing provides a number of benefits over other types of detox and cleansing diets. The liquid and fiber found in most high quality juices helps act as an appetite suppressant, preventing you from feeling hungry throughout the day. Unlike water fasts, juices provide some calories and plenty of nutrients, helping you avoid extreme tiredness. Juices can also improve your digestion and have even been shown to reduce total cholesterol over the course of the diet.

A short term juice fast is an excellent way to break bad habits and help you prepare your mind and body for a new, healthier way of living. It has been used to aid meditation and other relaxation techniques, especially when you combine it with travel or a retreat designed to reduce your overall stress levels. This kind of diet change can also help you shed excess water weight and clean out a sluggish digestive system, leaving you feeling fresher and lighter.

Juice diets aren't just for people who want dramatic changes, however. You can also use a modified version of many diet plans to help you include more fruit and vegetables in your diet, improve your caloric intake, or avoid unhealthy foods. Many juice recipes will help you get your recommended daily fruit and vegetable intake in just one drink. Juicing is a healthy choice that can work for almost everyone.

Getting the Nutrition You Need

Fruit and vegetable juices are nutrient-dense, but they also contain large amounts of water. That means you'll stay hydrated, but it can make it difficult to get the proper nutrition if you stick to just one or two types of juice. Many people take supplemental vitamins and herbal preparations while enjoying a juice fast to ensure that they won't suffer from any nutritional deficiencies.

You can also make a point of choosing juices that include the essential nutrients your body needs. For instance, green juices containing spinach can boost your iron intake, while broccoli can help you get the protein and calcium you need. Avocado provides many essential fats and can make your normal juices into delicious smoothies. While it might take a little while to get used to drinking your vegetables, all these juices can provide you with a great-tasting natural source of the vitamins and minerals you require.

Your Caloric Intake

Adding juice to your diet or using it to replace other foods can greatly affect your caloric intake. This can be beneficial if you're hoping to lose a little weight, but it's important to know what you're consuming. Sugar-heavy juices such as apple and orange contain a little more than 100 calories per cup. If you add that to your normal diet, you could find yourself gaining weight. Supplementing your normal food with juice is an excellent choice if you struggle with low bodyweight and have trouble eating enough, but it could cause problems if you're trying to lose weight instead of gaining.

Using juice as a meal replacement could cause the opposite problem if you don't monitor your intake. If you consume the same volume of juice as you would ordinary food, you may have trouble getting enough calories to keep your mood up and your body healthy. While replacing food with juice for a short period of time is a good idea if you want to lose a little, it can be disastrous if your intake drops too low.

Make sure you consume a larger volume during your juice fast than you would if you were eating normally. You'll feel better and your body will reward you with more energy. Drinking between 10 and 20 cups of fresh, delicious juice every day will help you meet your caloric needs and still lose weight. Just adjust the amount for your appetite and activity level.

Should You Try a Juice Diet?

While juice diets are a great choice for most people, they won't work for everyone. Doctors advise against using any kind of liquid diet if you are pregnant or nursing. This kind of diet is also usually a poor choice for children, people who have immune deficiencies, or anyone who normally suffers from fatigue or anemia. While these people can add juice to their diets for better health, doctors advise against even short term juice fasting.

If you suffer from hypoglycemia or diabetes, you may need to adjust a normal juice diet to accommodate your disorder. While this can feel like "cheating," it helps prevent strong fluctuations in blood sugar levels and ensures a healthier, safer cleansing process.

Modifying Juice Diets for Special Needs

If you consider yourself to be relatively healthy and aren't aware of any disorders or metabolic issues that might affect your diet, try a normal juice fast to start with. Don't afraid to adjust your diet if you experience dizziness, mood changes or feelings of excessive tiredness, however. You can add moderate amounts of fresh fruit, nuts or similar raw foods to your diet without causing problems.

If you are very active, you may also need to modify your juice diet to include low fat dairy or some meats. Just make sure you introduce these foods slowly and carefully, since they can interfere with the cleansing action of juice. If you're not sure how to modify your juice fast, talk to your doctor or nutritionist for professional advice. The best juice diet is the one you can sustain, after all.

Adding Juice to a Normal Diet

If you're not ready to try a juice-only fast, you can still get a lot of benefits by including juice in your normal diet. This is an especially good idea if you're tempted to skip meals or you know you have trouble consuming the amount of fresh vegetation your body needs to be healthy. Just make a glass of juice in the morning or evening and consume it instead of a meal or along with a light snack. The juice will help you avoid feeling hungry and will provide the nutrients you normally lack. It even works as a pick-me-up instead of chips or other unhealthy food in the afternoon.

Choosing a Juicer

If you're planning to make juice a major or the only component of your diet for any significant length of time, you won't be able to do your juicing by hand. A dedicated juicer provides you with better quality juice that contains more fiber and essential nutrients. It also makes it easier to produce green juices and beverages made from foods that are more difficult to juice by hand.

Because you need to be able to rely on your juicer, however, you can't just buy the first one with an appealing price tag. Dedicated juice fasters need high quality equipment to help them get the most out of nature's produce. The juicer you buy doesn't have to be extremely expensive, but it does need to be able to provide you with high quality, great-tasting juice, quickly and reliably.

Types – There are many different kinds of juicers available on the market, but some are too specialty for use during a juice diet. For instance, devices made primarily to extract citrus juices like orange or grapefruit may be handy for breakfast use, but they often fail to produce good results with vegetables and other fruits.

Look for an all-purpose juicer that works with every kind of ingredient you might want to juice.

Power – Many inexpensive juicers don't have the power you need to deal with whole fruits and vegetables. If your budget is limited and you're willing to pre-chop your food before juicing, you can go with a lower-powered model. If you want more convenience and more consistent juice, choose a more powerful device.

Size – A big juicer can handle more different kinds of fruits and vegetables without pre-chopping, but it might take up a lot of cabinet or counter space in your kitchen. If you live in a small apartment or another narrow space, choose compact models.

Ease of Use – Some juicers do a good job producing drinkable juice, but have to be fully disassembled for cleaning. If you'd like to make your juice quickly and easily, pick a model that's simple to clean. If you want a feature-filled device, you may have to sacrifice some simplicity.

Budget – Decide how much you can spend before you go shopping. It's possible to get a very basic but functional juicer for as little as $30 to $50. Top of the line juicers for people who want to include fresh fruit and veggie juices in their everyday lives cost more, up to several hundred dollars. In general, it's a good idea to choose a simple model from a well-regarded brand over a complex model from an unknown manufacturer when your budget is limited.

Feature Set – If you have limited space for appliances or want to perform more functions than just juicing, models with extra features could provide more bang for your buck. You can choose juicers that will also provide coconut milk, nut butter or other healthy homemade foods, but you may have to pay more.

Traveling with Juice

It's always best to consume your juices almost as soon as you make them, but that isn't always possible. After all, it can be very difficult to operate a juicer at the office. If you know you want to engage in a juice diet but you can't juice on the spot, store your finished drinks in durable, BPA-free containers such as glass or steel bottles. Most juices will keep for a few hours at room temperature or in the fridge, but don't do well after exposure to higher heat.

Fruit-Only Juices

When you hear about juice, you probably think about fruit. That's because these sweet, liquid-filled foods are a natural choice for juicing. Some fruits can be juiced using just a knife or reamer, but others require a little more care. Your electric juicer should be able to handle all kinds of delicious fruit, however.

Choose a variety of fresh specimens in their prime, avoiding fruit that seems dry and hard or which shows brown spots or has an over-ripe scent. Because fruit juices are so high in healthy natural sugars, they can be a great energy boost, but must be used in moderation by people with diabetes or glycemic problems.

Watermelon Cooler

This chilled watermelon beverage is the perfect healthy choice for a hot day. It's based on traditional agua frescas from Mexico and South America, but omits the unhealthy sugars often associated with these drinks.

Ingredients

4 cups cubed watermelon, seeds removed
10 to 12 ice cubes
3 limes

Place watermelon and ice into a powerful blender or food processor. Blend on high power until well combined. Juice the limes and add lime juice plus pulp to the watermelon mixture. Blend until slushy in texture. Pour into a tall glass and consume with a spoon or straw.

Apple Lemon Zinger

This recipe combines the sweet, crispness of fresh apples with the bright flavors of ginger and citrus. For best results, juice the apples with their skins. The result will be cloudier, but it also contains more fiber and important flavonoid compounds. Drink this beverage chilled, or warm it up for an excellent cold remedy. Avoid non-organic apples, which may have wax or pesticide residues on their skins.

Ingredients

2 fresh, sweet apples (Gala, Golden Russet, Jonagold and McIntosh work well)
1 medium lemon or lime
½ thumb-length of fresh ginger, or a piece about 1 inch square

Remove the seeds from the apples and chop if necessary. Peel the citrus fruit, setting aside the peelings for zest. Add all ingredients to your juicer or blender and process until the mixture is smooth and drinkable. If necessary, strain out the larger pieces, but this juice is best with all the fiber-rich pulp still in the mix.

Fresh Berry Medley

Berries are simple to juice and provide an extremely appealing color and flavor. They're also rich in antioxidants that have been associated with disease-fighting and anti-aging properties. Rinse your fruit carefully and choose only berries that are bright, plump and fragrant. Whenever possible, stick to locally-grown varieties that carry a lighter pesticide load and which have traveled shorter distances. They tend to be the freshest and healthiest option. You can substitute blackberries for the raspberries to produce a darker, tarter flavor.

Ingredients

2 cups blueberries
2 cups whole strawberries
2 cups red, black or yellow raspberries

Rinse all berries thoroughly to remove dust and chemical residues. Hull the strawberries, discarding the leaves. Place all the fruit into a juicer or blender and process until no fruit pieces are visible. The juice should be thick and opaque. If necessary, thin it with water until it reaches the desired consistency.

Sour Fruit Punch

This tart and refreshing recipe can really put some sparkle in your morning. It's the antidote to too-sweet commercial juices with added sweeteners. Dilute it with clear or sparkling water for a delicious spritzer or drink it straight for a juice that'll wake you up. You can reduce the acidity slightly by choosing pink grapefruit and Meyer lemons, or increase it with white grapefruit and Key limes. This juice is an excellent natural remedy for urinary problems, but it also makes a great day-to-day beverage.

Ingredients

2 juicing oranges, such as Navel, Valencia or Moro
1 medium grapefruit
1 Persian lime or two Key limes
1 medium lemon
1 ½ cups fresh red cranberries

Peel all the citrus fruits, setting the peels aside for later use as zest. Wash the cranberries thoroughly to remove dust and chemical residues. Place the peeled fruit and berries into your juicer or blender and process thoroughly. Strain to remove excess pulp if desired. Garnish with a thin strip of lemon zest and enjoy.

Strawberry Banana Smoothie

Strawberries and bananas are a classic combination that provides gentle sweetness and plenty of energy. The high carbohydrate content of the banana provides extra calories to help you keep going through the day, making this the perfect breakfast beverage or mid-afternoon juice snack. Look for fully-ripe yellow bananas to provide plenty of flavor. In fact, it's okay to use bananas with some spotting or browning in this recipe. Avoid green bananas, which can make the smoothie seem bitter or astringent.

Ingredients

1 ½ cups strawberries
1 large or 2 medium bananas
1 vanilla bean

Rinse and hull the strawberries, discarding the tops. Peel the banana and add both fruits to your blender or juicer, along with the vanilla bean. Process until the juice develops a thick, rich texture. The vanilla bean adds a sweet scent along with attractive tiny black flecks.

Tropical Starfruit Punch

Also called carambola, the starfruit is a tropical native from Southeast Asia. When ripe, it is soft, bright yellow and has a sweet-tart flavor that produces delicious juice. When combined with the unique flavor of fresh kiwi, this fruit truly shines, producing a memorable punch that makes an ideal breakfast beverage. Look for golden starfruit with smooth, thin skins and no brown spots, and tender kiwi with a fragrant smell. Avoid tired-looking fruits that seem soft or mushy. For a slightly sweeter flavor, choose mellow golden kiwi instead of the standard green variety.

Ingredients

3 starfruit
3 kiwi fruit

Wash both fruits and remove the fuzzy skins from the kiwis. Add all fruit to your blender or juicer and process until the entire mixture is smooth. If necessary, strain out any seeds or large pieces of pulp. Enjoy slowly over ice.

Mango Watermelon Juice

This sweet juice makes a great dessert beverage and provides most of the vitamins C and A you need in one day. Since watermelon is so high in moisture, you shouldn't need any additional water to produce a drinkable juice, but you can thin the result with sparkling water for a lighter drinking experience.

Ingredients

1 large mango
1 cup cubed watermelon

Peel and pit the mango, discarding all but the pulp. Cut the pulp into large cubes that will fit easily into your juicer. Remove all seeds from the watermelon. Process both fruits at once to produce an opaque, sunrise-colored juice.

Creamy Tropical Smoothie

Tropical flavors are appealing and traditional. They also make a great-tasting juice that's perfect as a breakfast beverage or quick snack. The extra carbohydrates from the banana provide this juice with more calories and energy potential than many other juice fast recipes. They also offer plenty of vitamin C, vitamin A and a little calcium.

Ingredients

1 mango
1 small banana
½ cup pineapple
½ cup papaya

Peel and pit the mango, discarding all but the pulp. Peel the banana. Cut the pineapple and the papaya into large cubes, removing seeds, core and skin. Add all ingredients to a powerful blender or juicer, adding water to achieve the desired thickness. Serve cold for best results.

Rich Berry Smoothie

This recipe is great for anyone whose juice fast includes dairy elements. It provides plenty of vitamins A, C and D, as well as calcium and protein. While the best berries are organic and local, you can use both fresh and frozen fruit. Look for low-fat yogurt from cows or goats that have received organic feed to reduce the possibility of chemical contamination. This smoothie is an excellent choice if you feel tired during your juice diet, and the natural cultures can help keep your digestive system healthy and happy.

2 sweet juicing oranges
1 large tart apple
¼ cup red or yellow raspberries
¼ cup strawberries
½ cup plain yogurt with live cultures

Peel the oranges and remove any seeds. Wash the apple and berries thoroughly. Hull the strawberries, discarding the leaves. Remove the seeds from the apple. Juice all fruits together and mix in the yogurt or add all ingredients to a blender and process until completely smooth.

Berry Mint Cooler

This drink is a great choice whenever you see fresh berries on sale and in season. The delicious natural sugars make this an excellent choice to provide a little bit of an energy boost first thing in the morning. Alternatively, add some ice and blend it with the juice to produce a delicious evening dessert or afternoon snack.

1 pound whole strawberries
2 cups fresh blackberries
2 cups fresh peppermint or spearmint
2 medium green kiwis

Wash all the fruit. Remove the peel from the kiwis and hull the strawberries, discarding the leaves. Pluck the mint leaves from their stems to reduce discoloration of this rich, purplish beverage. Process all ingredients together in a juicer with a large screen or a powerful blender. You'll be delighted by the sweetness that this juice has to offer.

Tropical Berry Treat

This quick recipe provides the great taste of tropical fruits combined with the tang of blackberries and the comforting flavor and texture of pear. You can enjoy it as is at breakfast, or try adding a few ice cubes in the blender for a bright-tasting smoothie you'll have again and again. The pears can make this drink a little grainy and opaque, but they provide a smooth background for all the other flavors, along with plenty of fiber.

Ingredients

3 medium green or golden kiwifruit
2 ripe Asian pears
¼ fresh pineapple
1 cup ripe blackberries

Peel the kiwifruit and pineapple. Remove the seeds and stem from the pears along with any core from your pineapple pieces. Place all the ingredients together in a blender and process until smooth. Serve chilled.

Tasty Cashew Shake

This recipe is a great choice for anyone who wants to keep more protein in their diet than most juice recipes offer. Adding a handful of raw nuts to your juice helps thicken it and can reduce cravings for natural fats and other important nutrients. Like other hearty juices, this beverage contains a few more calories than the average juice, but that doesn't make it a bad choice. Enjoy this recipe for dessert or as a quick pick-me-up.

Ingredients

½ cup whole raw cashews or almonds
¼ cup whole strawberries
1 small vanilla bean
½ teaspoon cinnamon
5 ice cubes

Soak the cashews for one hour in one cup of water to soften them and make them easier to blend. Hull the strawberries, discarding the leaves. Combine the cashews, their soaking water, and all other ingredients in a powerful blender on high. Process until the mixture is smooth and frothy.

Grapefruit Pineapple Splash

If you're on a grapefruit juice diet, you don't have to stick with boring beverages. This sparkling juice drink combines the great taste of pink grapefruit with tropical pineapple and a little bit of carbonated mineral water. Try this one to help you cool down on a hot summer day.

Ingredients

2 medium pink grapefruit
2 small pineapples
1 ½ cups sparkling water
5 ice cubes

Peel the grapefruit and pineapple, removing any seeds and the pineapple core. Chop the pineapple into large pieces. Put both fruits, the sparkling water and the ice cubes into a powerful blender. Process until the result is smooth and bubbly.

Green Juices

Green may not be the first color that comes to mind when you think about juice, but it should be an important part of any juicing diet. After all, green juices contain lots of important nutrients, antioxidants and other beneficial substances. While they may look a little unusual at first, their fresh, herbal flavor will soon make you a convert. If you're not sure you're ready for strongly-flavored green juices, try out recipes that include milder vegetables and herbs like parsley and cucumber. They'll help you prepare your taste buds for heartier combinations containing chard, kale and other leafy green nutritional powerhouses.

Basic Green Juice

This leafy green juice provides plenty of chlorophyll, plus a boost of iron, protein, calcium and other important nutrients. Celery, parsley and cucumber balance out the strong flavors of kale and spinach, providing a well-rounded taste and a great nutritional profile. Because leafy vegetables can be hard to process, use the celery and the cucumber to push them through your juicer.

Ingredients

2 cups spinach leaves
2 cups fresh parsley
1 cup kale
1 medium cucumber
1 stalk celery
Wash all vegetables thoroughly to remove dirt and chemical residues, even if they are organic in origin. Remove the parsley leaves from the stems and cut the stem end off of the cucumber. Add the first four ingredients to your blender or juicer and process until the liquid is smooth and has an even consistency. Add the cucumber and celery and process again. Enjoy this juice on its own or along with a light meal.

Bright and Spicy Green Juice

This green juice spices things up with a little hot pepper and ginger, providing interest, soothing upset stomachs, and keeping your immune system healthy. The spinach content is high enough to provide plenty of nutrition, but low enough to avoid a bitter flavor. For a different taste, try using Key limes or Meyer lemons instead of the standard varieties.

Ingredients

2 large cucumbers
2 cups spinach leaves
1 bunch fresh celery
1 bunch parsley
2 sweet apples, such as McIntosh
1 Persian lime or 2 Key limes
1 lemon
1 teaspoon ginger root
½ teaspoon red pepper

Wash all ingredients, removing the stem ends from the cucumbers and celery. Pluck the parsley leaves from their stems to prevent discoloration of the finished juice. Peel all citrus ingredients and remove the seeds from the apples. Add all the leafy ingredients to your juicer or blender, processing thoroughly, followed by the fruit, vegetable and spice ingredients. If necessary, strain to remove excess pieces of ginger or celery threads before consuming.

Ultimate Green Juice

This powerful green beverage contains some of the most nutrition-rich leafy greens available, combined with bright, fresh flavors that make it fun to drink. Because this juice can be a little thick, you may need to add some water during the juicing process. Alternatively, leave out the extra water and enjoy this drink as a green smoothie.

Ingredients

1 cup spinach leaves
4 large kale leaves
2 stalks celery
1 tart apple, such as Granny Smith
1 large cucumber
1 bunch cilantro
1 leaf green Swiss chard
½ lemon
fresh ginger to taste

Wash all ingredients thoroughly. Peel the lemon and remove the apple seeds. Pull the cilantro leaves from their stems to prevent discoloration of the final product. Process the leafy green ingredients first, fruit, spices and vegetables. Use the celery and cucumber to push any extra material into your juicer completely. Process the juice until the result is opaque, bright green, and free of lumps.

Neutral Green Juice

This variation on the basic green juice recipe provides a fairly neutral taste with a hint of mild sweetness. It's perfect for anyone who doesn't like strong or savory juices, as well as juice dieters who want a few more carbohydrates in their green beverages. Because the flavor of apples can vary significantly between varieties, pick one that provides the balance of sweetness and tartness that you prefer. Fuji, Golden Delicious and McIntosh are great places to start.

Ingredients

3 cups Romaine lettuce
2 cups kale
2 cups parsley
3 stalks celery
1 large cucumber
1 large sweet apple

Rinse all ingredients thoroughly to remove chemical residues and dirt. Pull the parsley leaves off of their stems and remove the seeds from the apple. Cut the stem end off of the cucumber. Add the leafy vegetables to your juicer or blender slowly, allowing them to process completely, followed by the apple, cucumber and celery stalks. Drink this juice as a mild start to your day or a calming before-bed treat.

Grapefruit Greens

This fruit and vegetable combo produces a healthy green juice with a tart citrus kick. Add a flavorful apple to the mix to provide some extra carbohydrates and a rounded sweetness that balances the sour and bitter citrus elements. This recipe produces a complex juice that will appeal to anyone who doesn't like their beverages to be simply sweet.

Ingredients

1 large bunch kale
4 stalks celery
1 large cucumber
1 white grapefruit
1 Persian lime or 2 Key limes
1 sweet apple, such as McIntosh, Gala or Honeycrisp

Remove all brown spots, insect damage and dirt or chemical residues from the ingredients. Cut the stem end off of the cucumber, remove the apple seeds and peel the citrus ingredients. Feed the kale leaves into the juicer one at a time, followed by the celery and cucumber. Add the fruit to the mixture slowly to produce a light green juice with a tart flavor.

Nopal Cactus Juice

Nopal cactus paddles, better known as prickly pear, are known for their ability to help balance blood sugar levels. These interesting vegetables also contain plenty of fiber to help keep your body healthy. To reduce the labor required to make this thick, smoothie-like beverage, choose cactus paddles that have already been de-spined. Use a blender or a juicer equipped with a large screen to preserve the thick, health-promoting pulp that this juice produces.

Ingredients

1 cups spinach leaves
1 medium cactus paddle
1 large tangerine
1 cup strawberries

Wash all ingredients and remove the spines from the cactus with pliers if necessary. Hull the strawberries, discarding the leaves, then peel the tangerine and remove any seeds. Blend or juice the spinach and cactus, adding water if necessary to keep the motor from laboring. Add the fruit, processing until there are no visible chunks and the mixture is smooth and thick.

Sweet Broccoli Juice

Tangerines add a little sweetness to this green juice, which provides plenty of vitamins C and K, along with phosphorus, B vitamins, manganese and magnesium. If you don't have access to tangerines, consider substituting a small orange or a Meyer lemon. The flavor will be slightly different, but the juice will still be delicious.

1 small head broccoli
4 stalks celery
2 tangerines
shredded ginger to taste

Peel the tangerines and remove any seeds. Wash the broccoli and celery, then process all ingredients until a smooth, thick juice is produced. Add water if desired and garnish with fresh ginger.

Pineapple Spinach Juice

Pineapple and spinach might seem like a strange combination, but they actually go together very well. This recipe provides calcium, iron and plenty of vitamins A and C. It can easily be made in a blender or a juicer, but it's best to use a large screen to capture all that delicious pineapple pulp.

Ingredients

1 cup fresh spinach
1 cup fresh pineapple
1 bunch parsley

Wash all ingredients and cut the pineapple into large pieces, trimming off the rind and core. Remove the parsley leaves from their stems to prevent discoloration of the juice. Put all ingredients into a blender or juicer, adding water to thin the mixture if necessary.

Spinach Fennel Drink

Fennel provides an exciting licorice taste to this sweet green juice. It's like having licorice candy in a healthy, refreshing drink. Like some other green juices, this one can look a little murky when it's finished, but the refreshing taste and smell make up for the look.

Ingredients

3 cups fresh spinach
2 large carrots
1 whole stalk fennel, bulb and leaves included
1 large tart apple

Remove the seeds from the apple and the stem ends from the carrots. Wash all the ingredients thoroughly. Cut the fennel into pieces that your blender or juicer can handle, then process the spinach, fennel and apple together. Use the carrots to push any remaining material through the juicer. Add a little extra water if the result is too thick for your preferences.

Green Lemonade

Lemonade is a lasting summer favorite, but conventional recipes include a lot of sugar and relatively little nutrition. This green lemonade recipe provides you with the powerful benefits of leafy green vegetables, plus the bright tang of lemon. A sweet apple and a little extra water help keep this tasty green beverage from being too sour.

1 cup kale
1 cup fresh spinach
2 stalks celery
1 large lemon
1 sweet red apple, such as Jonathan or Honeycrisp

Peel the lemon and remove any seeds from both it and the apple. Juice the leafy green vegetables, followed by the celery and the fruit. Dilute the finished juice with water to offset the tartness from the lemon, or add a small amount of natural sweetener such as agave nectar or honey.

Fruit and Vegetable Combinations

While fruit juices tend to outshine their humbler relatives, they can't always provide the same nutritional punch. That's why so many fruits are best combined with vegetables. These fruit and vegetable juice combinations add richness and greater energy potential to ordinary fruit flavors, producing a more complex and interesting beverage. While some of the ingredients may seem a little unusual, they don't negatively affect the flavor. You even might be surprised by how good these fruit and veggie juices can taste.

Rich and Creamy Breakfast Juice

If you want to be sure your body gets all the essential fats it needs, this juice is a great choice. It combines the health-giving properties of apples and carrots with the rich natural flavor of coconut and the brightness of ginger. You can substitute commercial canned coconut milk if fresh coconut isn't available, but make sure you choose a brand with no added water, gums or preservatives. This recipe is higher in calories than most other juices, so it's best enjoyed in moderation or when you expect to be active.

Ingredients

Meat from ½ large coconut or 1 small coconut
2 medium carrots
1 large sweet apple
½ inch fresh ginger

Grate the coconut using a hand grater or food processor. Add the grated coconut to a blender or juicer, along with about 1/3 cup water. Process until the mixture becomes very thick and the coconut is in many tiny pieces. Place the coconut and water mixture into your juicer using the fine screen. Run it through the juicer, allowing the screen to extract the coconut meat. You may need to remove the end piece to allow the coconut to pass through freely. Reserve the coconut meat for later use. Remove the seeds from the apple and add it to the juicer or a blender along with the carrots and ginger. Process until an opaque orange liquid is produced. Pour in 1/3 cup of fresh coconut milk, mixing thoroughly. Garnish with slivers of fresh ginger. For a thicker product, refrigerate the liquid first.

Berry Powerful Juice

Grapes and berries make a flavorful juice that supplies plenty of anti-oxidant compounds, but they can't provide all the nutrition your body needs. That's why combining them with fresh dark leafy greens such as kale or spinach is such a smart idea. These vegetables give you more energy and help you avoid running out of power midway through the day. They also combine well with the fruit, avoiding the bitter taste that sometimes comes with leafy greens alone.

Ingredients

2 cups blueberries or raspberries
2 cups red or Concord grapes
1 cup fresh kale
1 cup fresh spinach

Wash the fruit thoroughly. Remove the grapes from their stems and discard the stems. Remove any wilted or yellow leaves from the kale and spinach. Process all the fruit and vegetables in a juicer or powerful blender, adding water if necessary. Chill and drink along with a light snack. Add 2 tablespoons of your favorite protein powder for a meal replacement drink.

Nutritious Peach Juice

Fresh summer peaches are a sweet, sticky favorite for many people, but they get even better on a foundation of powerful, nutritious green vegetables. This flavorful juice includes strong-tasting fruits that effectively cover the taste of nutrition-packed greens like broccoli and spinach. While the color of this juice recipe might be a little surprising, the flavor and nutrient profile simply can't be beat. Try it on its own, or as a quick vitamin shot along with an ordinary meal. Using only the broccoli stalks allows you to reserve the more-tender florets for use in salads or other healthy recipes.

Ingredients

3 ripe peaches
1 tart apple
2 stalks broccoli
1 cup spinach leaves

Wash all fruits and vegetables thoroughly. Remove the tough ends of the broccoli, the pits from the peaches, and the seeds from the apples. Place all ingredients in a blender or juicer and process until smooth. The result may be slightly brownish in color, but the flavor will be all fruit.

Mint Wake-Up Call

While the name suggests a breakfast juice, you can enjoy this refreshing recipe at any time of the day. This juice combines morning staples like grapefruit and orange with hearty carrots and light-tasting celery. Topped off with the cool, bright taste of mint, this juice makes a great start to the day or an excellent choice to brighten up a slow evening. Use a large screen in your juicer to ensure you get plenty of fiber in your juice.

Ingredients

2 juicing oranges (Valencia works well)
1 medium pink or white grapefruit
1 large carrot
1 stalk green celery
½ cup peppermint or spearmint leaves

Wash the celery and carrot, removing all grit. Remove the leaves from the mint stems to keep the color of the finished product consistent. Peel the citrus. Combine all ingredients in the juicer, adding the mint before the carrot. Use the carrot to push the leafy material through the juicer.

Serve over ice.

Spicy Orange Pineapple

Orange and pineapple are a classic combination, but on their own they can be overpowering. That's why this hearty juice includes lime, carrots and chili. The more complex flavor is sure to be a winner at your table. Plus, your body will appreciate the vitamin C, pineapple enzymes and metabolism-boosting capsaicin. To produce a crisp smoothie, add a few ice cubes to the mixture in a blender.

Ingredients

2 sweet juicing oranges, such as Valencia or Moro
1 medium carrot
1 cup chopped pineapple
1 lime
1 small red pepper

Peel the citrus fruits and remove any seeds. Wash the carrot and remove any core or peel from the pineapple. Combine all ingredients in a blender or juicer with enough water to produce a smooth, drinkable consistency.

Ginger Pear Juice

Pears and ginger are another classic combination that's found in crisps, ciders and a range of other foods. While these dishes might not be right for a juice fast, the basic flavor is. Pears provide plenty of fiber, while ginger helps promote healthy digestion, making this an excellent juice for anyone who has recently overindulged.

Ingredients

1 medium pear
1 stalk celery
1 tablespoon fresh ginger

Wash all ingredients and remove the stem and seeds from the pear. Combine the fruit and ginger in a blender or juicer, processing until smooth. For a creamier texture, add a few ice cubes.

Spicy Apple Lemonade

This flavorful fruit juice includes a sweet yellow pepper to boost its nutritional value. You'll enjoy the cleansing effects of this beverage, as well as its mild, pleasant flavor. To increase tartness, simply add another lemon to the mix.

Ingredients

3 large sweet apples, such as Fuji
1 lemon
1 sweet yellow bell pepper
1 tablespoon ginger

Peel the lemon and remove any seeds. Wash the pepper and apples thoroughly to get rid of dirt and chemical residues. Seed all the apples and remove the seeds, stem and interior ribs from the pepper. Add all ingredients to a powerful blender or a juicer with a large screen and process until smooth. Drink chilled.

Red Summer Cooler

This interesting juice fast recipe combines the classic pairing of tomatoes and basil with sweet red strawberries. The best berries are organic, local and in season, but if these aren't available you can choose fragrant berries and wash them well. Garnish the finished juice with mint for greater complexity and even more great phytonutrients.

Ingredients

1 pound ripe red tomatoes
½ pound whole strawberries
5 leaves sweet basil

Hull the strawberries and tomatoes, discarding the leaves. If necessary, cut the tomatoes into pieces your juicer is able to handle. Process the fruit and basil leaves together to produce a strikingly red, flavorful beverage. Serve over ice.

Vegetable Citrus Medley

This drink is rich in a variety of vitamins, minerals and phytonutrients. While it uses vegetables more usually associated with soups and stews, that shouldn't put you off. The result is a complex beverage with an unusual color and plenty of health-promoting properties.

Ingredients

2 large juicing oranges
1 medium carrot
1 small lemon
1 stalk celery
½ cup raw red beets
½ cup spinach leaves

Peel the citrus fruits and remove any seeds. Wash the greens and other vegetables thoroughly. Process the lemon and oranges first, followed by the leafy greens. Use the celery and carrots to push any leftover material through your juicer. Serve over ice with ginger if desired.

Apple Squash Dessert Juice

One of the biggest problems for many juice dieters is the difficulty of finding a satisfying dessert juice. After all, juice may be exciting and refreshing, but it's hard to measure up to cake and ice cream. This recipe offers some of the same flavors you'll find in a good, natural apple pie, including the spicy zip of cinnamon. That's why it's such a great choice for anyone who craves dessert but prefers a healthy option.

Ingredients

1 medium butternut squash (about 1 ½ pounds)
4 medium sweet apples, such as Honeycrisp
1 teaspoon ground cinnamon

Wash the apples and squash to remove dirt and chemical residues. Slice the squash in half, remove the seeds, and cut the flesh into large cubes. De-seed the apple and remove its stem. Run the apple and the squash cubes through your blender or juicer, adding water as necessary. Stir in the cinnamon and garnish with a cinnamon stick if desired. Drink this enjoyable dessert beverage chilled or warmed.

Asian-inspired Citrus Cabbage Blend

Cabbage gets a bad reputation with many people due to its tendency to become sulfurous and bitter when overcooked. Fresh cabbage has a crisp texture and zesty flavor that makes it the star of some unusual salads as well as this delightful juice. The combination of tropical citrus, Asian pears and other Chinese ingredients will make this one of your favorite lunch or dinner-time juices.

Ingredients

1 small head bok choy, napa or green cabbage
3 medium carrots
2 tart green apples
2 Persian limes
1 lemon
1 Asian pear
1 thumb-length of ginger

Peel the lemon and limes. Wash the cabbage, carrots, pear and apples thoroughly. Remove the seeds and stems from the apples and pear. Cut off the stem end from the carrots and chop the cabbage into manageable chunks. Process all the ingredients in a juicer or blender, starting and finishing with an apple. Pour over ice and drink quickly.

Hunger-Defeating Smoothie

Especially when you're in the middle of a longer juice fast, hunger can creep up when you least expect it. If you want to defeat that growling monster without breaking your diet, this smoothie could be the perfect answer. By including avocado and banana with more conventional juice ingredients like mango, it offers more calories and an increase in energy. Use this juice sparingly, when you know you'll need more fuel than usual.

Ingredients

1 large banana
1 mango
1 large green avocado, such as Bacon or Zutano
10 to 12 ice cubes
1 teaspoon cumin

Peel and seed the avocado and the mango, reserving only the pulp. Cut all fruit ingredients into chunks and place in a powerful blender with the ice cubes. Puree until completely smooth, adding water to adjust the texture. Serve in a large glass.

Hearty Sweet Potato

Sweet potatoes may seem like an unlikely choice for juice, but they provide a starchy heartiness that can give you an extra boost in the middle of the day. Their mild flavor combines well with the mellow carrots, peppers and apples in this recipe, while tangerines offer a little bit of sweetness. In addition to a great taste, this juice provides plenty of vitamin A and folate.

Ingredients

3 sweet tangerines
2 sweet golden apples, such as Golden Delicious
2 large carrots
1 medium raw sweet potato
1 medium sweet red pepper

Peel the tangerines and remove any seeds. Wash all the other ingredients thoroughly. Cut off the stem ends of the carrots and pepper, removing the seeds and ribs from the pepper. Remove the stem and seeds from the apples and peel the sweet potato, cutting it into large cubes. Process all of the ingredients in a powerful blender or juicer, saving one tangerine for last.

Festive Fruit and Vegetable Juice

This juice includes all kinds of nutritious and colorful fruits and vegetables in a delicious mixture. It'll help you increase your intake of all those important dietary elements without any trouble. If you choose to use the beet greens, choose younger specimens with a milder flavor.

Ingredients

4 medium carrots
4 large Brussels sprouts
2 ripe yellow pears
2 sweet red apples
1 medium beet, with or without greens
1 ripe red tomato
2 leaves arugula
½ small head cauliflower
½ small head broccoli
¼ ripe pineapple

Wash all the ingredients thoroughly. Trim off the stem and root ends of the beet and carrots. Remove all the seeds from the apples and pears. Peel the pineapple and remove the core. Juice all ingredients, adding the broccoli, cauliflower, arugula and beet greens along with wetter ingredients such as apples and carrots. Thin with water as desired and drink at room temperature.

Slim Summer Cooler

This fresh juice is full of slender cucumbers and celery, both of which act as natural diuretics to help your body flush out more water. It also contains bright, flavorful apples, ginger and lime. The result is light, refreshing and delightful.

Ingredients

1 large sweet pink apple, such as Pink Lady
1 small cucumber
1 stalk celery
½ Persian lime or 1 Key Lime
5 ice cubes
1 teaspoon fresh ginger

Rinse all the ingredients. Remove the stems from the cucumber and apple, along with the apple seeds. Process all ingredients in a powerful blender to produce a smooth, creamy slush with a bright flavor. Serve immediately.

Savory Juices

Most juice diet recipes are fruit-based and tend to be fairly sweet, but not everyone wants to consume sweet food and drinks all the time. If you're not all that fond of sweets, you might find that many juice fast recipes are too cloying for your tastes. That's why this book includes a set of delicious savory juice recipes. While they include some fruit, they provide a set of additional, more interesting flavors that can add a little dimension to your juice diet plan. While some of the combinations may seem intimidating at first, they're sure to grow on you.

Jugo de Pepino

This cool, cucumber-based recipe offers a fresh flavor with only the smallest hint of sweetness. Limes and fresh cilantro provide a bright flavor, and fresh peppers give it a hint of spice. If you'd like to bring up the heat, consider substituting serrano or jalapeno peppers for the poblano. For a milder flavor, use a fresh green bell pepper or a Spanish frying pepper. Leave the stems on the cilantro for the best nutritional profile or remove them to produce a more appealing color.

Ingredients

3 medium cucumbers
2 large bunches cilantro
1 large poblano pepper
1 Persian lime or 2 Key limes
2 tart apples (Granny Smith works well)

Wash all fruits and vegetables thoroughly. Peel the lime and remove the seeds from the apples. Cut the stems, seeds and ribs out of the pepper. Wash your hands thoroughly, especially if you use spicy peppers. Place the apples, pepper and lime in the juicer and process. Add the cilantro, followed by the cucumbers. If necessary, use a cucumber to push the leafy parts of the cilantro

through the juicer. Chill and dilute if desired or serve
immediately over ice.

Autumn Squash Delight

Multiple kinds of squash provide a rich, velvety texture and subtle flavor in this thick, hearty juice that's just right for autumn. Choose brightly-colored vegetables with smooth, firm skins and a hollow sound. Avoid any specimen with dark spots or soft areas, which can indicate rot. To spice things up, add a cinnamon stick or a pinch of nutmeg to the finished product. It's the perfect option for anyone who loves autumn vegetables but doesn't want the overly-sweet taste of dessert.

1 small pie pumpkin
1 medium butternut or acorn squash
2 medium carrots
2 yellow crookneck squash

Wash all vegetables thoroughly, removing stems. Remove the seeds from the pumpkin and winter squash, chopping them into pieces small enough to fit into your juicer or blender. Combine all the ingredients in the juicer, adding water periodically until you produce a rich, smoothie-like puree. Pour into a tall glass or enjoy with a spoon.

Spicy Immune Booster

This unusual combination of ingredients could help you fight off an oncoming cold or get over an existing one. Since the flavors are very strong, you may wish to dilute the drink with water. Alternatively, you can drink it all at once as a "shot." While this juice recipe may not seem appealing at first, your immune system will thank you.

Ingredients

1 medium lemon, 2 Persian limes or 3 to 4 Key limes
2 cloves garlic or 1 clove elephant garlic
1 small Cayenne pepper

Peel the citrus fruit and garlic cloves. Add all the ingredients to a juicer or blender and process until smooth, using a large screen to allow pulp to pass through. Add a few tablespoons of water if necessary to liquefy the result. Thin with water or drink quickly for a boost to your immune system.

Rich Tomato Juice

Tomato juice is a classic choice for people who don't like sweets but prefer to drink their fruits and vegetables. Plain tomato beverages can lack an interesting flavor and nutrition profile, however. That's why this recipe adds classic tomato accompaniments like spinach, garlic, basil, peppers and chili. The result is a fresh, tasty beverage that gives you all the tastes of your favorite bruschetta topping.

Ingredients

10 ripe plum tomatoes
1 cup spinach leaves
1 sweet bell pepper
20 leaves basil
2 small cloves garlic
1 small red chili

Rinse all ingredients except garlic. Remove the stem ends from the tomatoes, bell pepper and chili. Peel the garlic cloves. De-seed the peppers and remove the internal ribs. Wash your hands after handling the chili pepper. Process all the ingredients through a blender or juicer, starting with the first 8 tomatoes and finishing with the last two tomatoes to remove pepper residue from the juicer. Drink hot or cold.

Creamy Avocado Carrot Smoothie

Smoothies don't all have to be sticky-sweet concoctions. The inclusion of avocado in this recipe gives it a rich, satisfying taste with plenty of the beneficial fats you need to fight hunger and fuel a busy day. The cumin provides depth and interest that many other smoothies lack. For variety, add a little water and consume this recipe as a chilled soup.

2 large carrots
1 small, black avocado such as Hass or Lamb Hass
1 fresh scallion
½ teaspoon ground cumin or cumin seed

Wash the carrots and scallion, removing the stem end of the carrot and the roots and any damaged leaves from the onion. Juice both vegetables, thinning the end product until you have about 1 cup of juice. Remove the skin and the seed from the avocado and add it to a blender along with the juice and the cumin. Process the mixture until it is smooth and creamy. Serve chilled or at room temperature.

Salsa Verde Juice

This spicy juice will remind you of some of the best Central American salsas. To increase the heat, choose a spicier pepper such as serrano. To reduce the spiciness, substitute poblano or other mild peppers, but try it out at full strength first. The avocado in this recipe counteracts much of the heat, producing a delicious savory drink that you'll love.

Ingredients

2 medium green bell or Italian frying peppers
5 medium tomatillos
1 small avocado
1 medium bunch cilantro
2 whole scallions
1 small jalapeno pepper
1 teaspoon cumin
1 small clove garlic

Wash the peppers, tomatillos, cilantro, scallions and pepper. Remove the stems, seeds and ribs from all the peppers, washing your hands after handling any chilies. De-seed and peel the avocado, reserving the pulp only. Tear the papery shells off of the tomatillos and the garlic. Remove all cilantro leaves from their stems to prevent discoloration of the juice and discard the stems. Process all ingredients but the avocado in a juicer or blender. Remove ¼ cup of juice from the recipe and mash it with the avocado. Return the avocado mixture to the main recipe and process until completely smooth. If desired, serve with a wedge of lime.

Vegetable Crudites

If you love fresh, raw vegetables as a snack, this juice will be perfect for you. It includes all your favorite dipping veggies, along with a handful of exciting herbs. You won't even miss the dip! If fresh dill is not available, you can substitute dried dill weed or dill seeds for a slightly different result.

1 small head cauliflower
1 small stalk broccoli, including the stem
6 medium carrots
3 large stalks celery
1 tablespoon fresh dill

Rinse all the ingredients thoroughly to remove any dirt or chemical residues. Chop the broccoli and cauliflower into manageable pieces. Process all the ingredients in a juicer or powerful blender until completely smooth. Add water if necessary to achieve the desired texture.

Souper Italian Juice

This smooth beverage has just a little bit of sweetness, like your favorite red sauce or a good vegetable soup. If you'd like a slightly stronger flavor, add a little hot sauce or some Italian seasoning to the vegetables when you process them. This can be served cold as a juice or warm as a soup.

Ingredients

1 ½ pounds large ripe tomatoes
¾ pound spinach
¾ pound medium carrots
1 sweet yellow pepper
1 sweet red pepper
1 sweet orange pepper
1 small stalk celery
1 medium bunch flat-leaf Italian parsley

Wash all the ingredients. Remove the stems, seeds and internal ribs from the peppers and cut off the stem ends of the carrots. Process all the ingredients in a blender or juicer, starting with the leafy ingredients and finishing with the celery. Pour into a tall glass or a bowl and enjoy.

Homemade V-8

This recipe doesn't include the same vegetable mix as the original V-8, but unlike its commercial cousin, it's uncooked and won't expose you to hazardous chemicals from can and bottle linings. Use fresh, organically-produced ingredients with no dark or soft spots for best results.

Ingredients

1 pound large ripe tomatoes
½ pound fresh spinach
½ pound large carrots
1 small beet
1 stalk celery
1 whole green onion
1 small bunch Italian flat-leaf parsley
1 small head leaf lettuce

Remove the stem ends from the beet, carrots and lettuce. Wash all vegetables thoroughly, separating the lettuce leaves from the main bunch. Process all the leafy vegetables through a juicer or powerful blender, followed by the beet, tomatoes, carrots, onion and celery. The result is hearty, healthy and satisfying.

Eggplant Delight

If eggplants and collard greens sound like a strange choice for a beverage, they shouldn't. The complex taste of the many vegetables in this drink provide a well-rounded, soup-like flavor that makes a great choice for lunch or dinner. Because this recipe uses a small amount of many different veggies, it's an excellent choice for using up leftover
ingredients. Feel free to alter this recipe according to the food you have on hand.

Ingredients

½ pound romaine lettuce
¼ pound collard greens
¼ pound carrots
¼ pound cauliflower florets
1 tiny eggplant
1 small sweet green pepper
1 small sweet yellow pepper
1 small sweet red pepper
1 stalk celery
1 small tomato
black pepper to taste

Wash all the ingredients thoroughly. Remove the stems

from the peppers and carrots. Cut out the seeds and ribs from the peppers and discard them. Juice all ingredients in a blender or high quality juicer, reserving the celery stick to push through any remaining material. Drink immediately.

Spicy Orange Drink

This recipe produces a brilliant orange beverage with a hint of natural sweetness that's balanced by the bright flavors of tomato and a little bit of spice. Garnish with ½ teaspoon of hot sauce and some freshly ground black pepper for a beautiful and delicious treat.

Ingredients

¾ pound tomatoes
2 medium sweet red peppers
2 medium sweet yellow peppers
6 medium carrots
½ teaspoon black pepper

Remove the stems, seeds and ribs from the peppers and cut off the stem end of all the carrots. Wash all the vegetables thoroughly. Process the vegetable ingredients, starting with the tomatoes and finishing with the carrots. Mix in ½ teaspoon of black pepper and garnish as desired. Enjoy the result at room temperature.

Gazpacho Juice

This savory juice is reminiscent of gazpacho, the classic Mediterranean summer soup. Like traditional gazpacho, it's mean to be served cool, but unlike its ancestor, this drink is uncooked and full of great nutrients.

6 medium tomatoes
4 stalks celery
1 medium sweet red pepper
1 medium cucumber
1 small bunch cilantro
1 small red onion

Peel the onion. Wash all the other ingredients and remove the cilantro leaves from their stems to prevent discoloration of the finished juice. Process all the ingredients in a blender or juicer, starting with the tomatoes and finishing with the celery. Serve slightly chilled.

Creamy Romaine Blend

This vegetable-based drink is surprising light and creamy in flavor. Some testers even compared it to a cream soda. You'll be surprised by how addictive this lettuce-based juice can be.

¾ pound Romaine lettuce or one whole Romaine heart
1 medium sweet orange pepper
1 celery heart
1 large cucumber
Peel the cucumber. Wash all other ingredients, breaking the lettuce and celery heart down into leaves and stalks. Remove the stem, seeds and internal ribs from the pepper. Combine all the ingredients in a juicer or blender, using one celery stalk to push through any extra material. Drink chilled or at room temperature.

No-Tomato Red Juice

This bright red juice looks as though it should be chock full of tomatoes, but the flavor is both milder and more sharp. This rich, attractive drink will soon become a summer favorite at your house.

1 small bunch spinach
4 large stalks celery
1 medium beet
1 small bunch parsley
1 medium sweet red pepper
2 small red radishes
2 medium cucumbers

Peel the cucumbers, remove the stem and root ends from the beet, and cut out the stem, seeds and ribs from the pepper. Remove the tops from the radishes and set aside for other recipes. Wash all ingredients thoroughly, then process in a juicer or blender until you produce an opaque, startlingly red juice. Drink slightly chilled or over ice.

Basic Savory Juice

This relatively simple savory drink works well on its own or as a base for other juices. It also helps provide some of the sodium that many juice diets lack. While this recipe produces a raw juice, the flavor is fairly close to that of vegetable broth, making it a hydrating and satisfying option.

Ingredients

1 bunch celery
3 pounds ripe red tomatoes
1 small head leaf lettuce
salt to taste

Wash all the ingredients carefully and remove the stem end from the celery. Feed the vegetables into the juicer, starting with the tomatoes and finishing with the celery. Salt and add water according to your preferences. This juice can be consumed warm, cold or at room temperature.

Sample Juice Diet Meal Plans

A Three Day Juice Diet

The three juice diet or "juice fast" is a popular choice for people who want to cleanse their bodies periodically, as well as those who are new to juice fasting. This diet gives your digestive system a bit of a break while washing out all the built-up toxins and other substances that sometimes come from a standard Western diet. This sample meal plan will help you develop your preferred juice regimen, but it's only an example. Feel free to change it according to what works best for you.

Day 1:

Breakfast – Strawberry Banana Smoothie
Mid-morning Snack – Vegetable Citrus Medley
Lunch – Eggplant Delight
Afternoon Snack – Mango Watermelon Juice
Dinner – Bright and Spicy Green Juice
Dessert – Berry Mint Cooler

Day 2:

Breakfast – Tropical Starfruit Punch
Mid-morning Snack – Berry Powerful Juice
Lunch – Hearty Sweet Potato
Afternoon Snack – Vegetable Crudites
Dinner – Homemade V-8
Dessert – Spicy Apple Lemonade

Day 3:
Breakfast – Rich and Creamy Breakfast Juice
Mid-morning Snack – Basic Savory Juice
Lunch – Hunger-Defeating Smoothie
Afternoon Snack – Gazpacho Juice
Dinner – Creamy Romaine Blend
Dessert – Tasty Cashew Shake

Remember to drink a glass of water before consuming each juice to help promote good digestion. Drink juices slowly, don't gulp them, and make your dessert beverage one you drink three or more hours before you sleep. There's no strict limit to how much juice you should drink. Just remember that the average juice contains about 100 calories per eight ounce glass, and you need about 1,000 calories per day even on a very strict diet. If you're more active, just increase the amount you consume.

The 10 Day Juice Diet

Juice diets can be extended for five, seven and up to 10 days without significant modifications. It is more important to pay attention to your nutrition levels and fiber consumption when you go on a longer juice fast, however. Because you won't be returning to normal food as quickly, your body will need plenty of support to ensure good health and proper cleansing. If you've never done a juice diet before, start with a shorter period, then work your way up.

Because 10 day juice diets require different things from different people, a strict plan isn't necessarily appropriate. Instead, we recommend consuming specific types of juices at various points throughout the day. You can vary the exact choices you make, as long as you stick to the same general juice types. That'll give you a more interesting diet over the course of your juice fast, as well as greater control over what you take in.

Breakfast – A sweet fruit-based juice with plenty of natural sugars to help you get started. Try a Tasty Cashew Shake, a Rich and Creamy Breakfast Juice, or a Tropical Berry Treat to get you ready for the day.

Mid-morning Snack – In the middle of the morning, a light but interesting juice can help you keep going. Consider having No-Tomato Red Juice, Bright and Spice Green Juice, or Salsa Verde Juice to pep things up.

Lunch – Most people want something savory for lunch, with enough energy potential to see them through the afternoon. Eggplant Delight and Asian-inspired Citrus Cabbage Blend are both excellent choices.

Afternoon Snack – If you suffer from the afternoon doldrums, you need a carbohydrate boost. The right juices, such as a Strawberry Banana Smoothie, Nopal Cactus Juice, or Autumn Squash Delight, will provide that boost and keep your mood and energy levels up. If you tend to feel hungry, focus on choices that include banana, avocado or coconut.

Dinner – The best juices for evening are savory and relatively light, but complex enough to satisfy. Creamy Romaine Blend, Spicy Orange Drink, Jugo de Pepino, or Rich Tomato Juice are all great choices. Green juices like Spinach Fennel Drink and Grapefruit Greens can also be an excellent choice.

Dessert – Dessert juices can be something of an indulgence, whether they contain mostly sweet fruit or a little extra fat. Try Mango Watermelon Juice, Apple Squash Dessert Juice, or a smoothie a few hours before bed. It'll help you avoid craving less beneficial food and will give you something to look forward to.

In addition to these beverages, you can add green juices throughout the day, as well as chia, ground flax, hemp powder, spirulina or legume protein. These additives can thicken up a disappointing juice and help you feel more full. They also provide a number of nutrients that you don't find in apples or kale. The key is to ensure plenty of variety.

Never engage in a 10 day juice diet that contains the same few recipes day after day. It's sure to get boring and it could counteract some of the benefits that are normally associated with drinking these healthy fruit and vegetable juices. Remember to drink water throughout the day, as well; juice is full of liquid, but it doesn't fully replace water.

Breaking Your Juice Fast

It can be tempting to dive right into normal food after a juice fast, but this not only goes against the spirit of the diet, it could also cause you harm. Because your stomach is primarily used to plant foods and minimal bulk after a fast, you need to work your way up to regular eating. For the first day, stick to fresh vegetables, fruit, nuts, light soups and plant oils. The second day, try adding some whole grains, such as brown rice, or cooked starchy vegetables and beans.

Wait until day three or four to reintroduce dairy to your diet, and stick to very small amounts at first. This will keep you from feeling bloated or suffering from digestive problems while your body remembers how to deal with solid foods. Pay attention to how you feel when you introduce new foods; if you become uncomfortable or have a strong reaction, your body may be trying to tell you something.

Juice Dieting for Longer Periods

Even well-planned juice diets tend to be very low in calories. They also provide your body with relatively little protein and fat. While this can be extremely beneficial in the short term, many people have trouble using a juice diet for longer periods. While some people have stuck to only juice for as long as 60 or 90 days, this is something you shouldn't do without a lot of careful planning.

If you find that you love juice dieting, consider talking to a nutritionist about the best way to get what your body needs on juice alone. Alternatively, just limit your daily consumption of solid food a little and add in more juice. You'll get many of the same benefits you encounter with fasting, but experience less strain on your body.

Conclusion:

When you do it right, juice dieting can offer a lot of health benefits. It'll clean out potentially dangerous dietary toxins, help you reduce bloating and discomfort, and restart your body after a period of poor health choices. While no diet can work miracles, one based on plenty of fresh fruits and vegetables provides an excellent way to lose a few pounds and feel a lot better. Try out a few tasty juice recipes today; you'll soon be excited by the prospect of drinking these delicious, healthy juices and enjoying a lighter, more energized life. If you've never spent much time thinking about the benefits of juice, it's time to get started.

Lightning Source UK Ltd.
Milton Keynes UK
UKOW05f1820010217
293402UK00022B/563/P

9 781630 228866